"Listen to Me, Doctor"

"Listen to Me, Doctor"

Taking Charge of Your Own Health Care

Marti Ann Schwartz

The Consummate Consumer™

MacMurray & Beck

ASPEN, COLORADO

Printed and bound in the United States of America

Library of Congress Cataloging-in-Publication Data
Schwartz, Marti Ann, 1955–
    "Listen to me, Doctor" : taking charge of your own health care /
Marti Ann Schwartz.
        p.   cm.
    ISBN 1-878448-67-6
    I. Medical care.   2. Consumer education.   I. Title.
RA410.5.S34   1995
362.1—dc20   95-18654
                                                                  CIP

Book design by Jody Chapel.
The text was set in Garamond by Pro Production.

Publisher's disclaimer

Both the publisher and the author assert here that no one
under any form of medical care or maintenance should
alter his or her regimen without thoroughly discussing
any change in diet or medication with a qualified physician.

**This book is dedicated
with love and gratitude to:**

My Dad and Mom—They gave me life, and although dismayed at times
by the choices I've made, have been my most vocal supporters.

And most of all, to my husband, Ken, and daughter, Erin.
Ken, our life together hasn't always been easy, but
you've got to admit it has *never* been dull!
And Erin . . . I would never have chosen the journey I went through,
but having you in my life has made it worthwhile!

Contents

Chapter 3

The Doctor–Health-Care Consumer Team 27

Chapter 4

Finding a New and Better Doctor. 41

Chapter 9

Senior Health Care. 123

Chapter 10

Children's Health Care. 139

Preface

In January 1990, I was five months pregnant with my first child and I was diagnosed with Hodgkin's disease, a form of cancer.

I never had had a positive attitude toward the health-care community before this crisis, and my feelings didn't change as my pregnancy continued. I was given diagnostic tests by lab technicians who were far more interested in the outcome of the tests than in my well-being or that of my baby. In fact, my pregnancy seemed quite an inconvenience for everyone except me and my husband. The one mention of my pregnancy was made by a nurse in the hospital when I had a biopsy. She couldn't understand why I wasn't happy and *glowing*.

In the past I had been able to avoid going to doctors. Now I had no choice. I was desperate to know what was happening to me and what I could do about it. That's when I became a health-care consumer. I found out how to get what I needed from my doctors and the health-care system.

It wasn't long before friends, family, and even people I hardly knew began asking for my help in dealing with doctors, hospitals, and medical issues in general. I gave seminars to groups, showing others how to deal with the health-care maze. It is a subject that affects everyone—young and old, men and women, the sick *and* the healthy! I was urged to write a book and share my experience and knowledge with others. Then I talked to a few of my doctors. They thought it was a great idea, especially since most doctors are uncomfortable with the common belief that "doctors have all the answers." They would prefer, they told me, to emphasize the teamwork that comes from working with informed patients.

This book is not just for those who are sick or those involved with others who are sick. It is for everyone who wants to learn how to get quality health care.

I will show you how to find the right health-care providers for you, and I'll discuss the health-care environment in general. In this book you will learn money-saving tips, how to deal with health insurance companies and Medicare, and about the variety of health insurance programs offered. I will also discuss specific health-care concerns for men, women, seniors, and children. After reading this book, you'll know what to ask for and who to ask.

Many people are great consumers in other areas of their lives, but they don't use a consumer's approach when dealing with the health-care community. Medicine is the biggest business in America and all normal business practices apply, including the rights of the consumer. I have seen what happens when you stand up for those rights. My first experience as a consumer with health care was in college, when a five-minute medical visit resulted in a $350 bill. I called to complain and the doctor reduced the charges.

If you approach the health-care community as the business it is, you'll be able to stand up for your rights as a consumer. Don't allow others to decide what is best for you.

Marti Ann Schwartz

Acknowledgments

The content of this book is based on interviews with doctors and nurses, hospital administrators, health insurance executives, medical association personnel, and many others who work in the medical field. Experiences described throughout the book were provided by my seminar attendees. I thank you all for your honesty and candor.

I have been fortunate to have the support of truly exceptional doctors. Dr. Robert Goldman helped me deal with the medical aspects of cancer as well as the fear, anger, and pain that came with it. He was a loving, compassionate doctor and he will be sorely missed. Dr. Larry Veltman is proof that when looking for a second opinion, sometimes you end up with a better doctor. He walks on water! In addition to overseeing my care and the healthy delivery of my daughter, he helped confirm the healthcare decisions made during my pregnancy.

I value the continuing support of my brother, Brian. It helps to have a marketing consultant in the family! His business insight has been as welcome as his helpful tips in dealing with the wonderful world of medicine.

And Debbie Scott, your wisdom has been invaluable. Thank you for your friendship. I treasure it.

M.A.S.

Chapter 1

The Rules of the Game

My Uncle Harry told me life was a game. No matter how bad things got or how many times I got knocked down, he said, it was my job to keep getting up again or I would lose the game. When I was diagnosed with cancer during my first pregnancy, the stakes of the game were raised. No longer was I responsible for just my own survival, I also had to ensure the well-being of my baby. Any decisions I made put two lives at risk.

I was most frustrated at not having control of my life. No one likes being told what to do or when and how to do it. The doctors wanted to do just that. They were used to deciding on treatment plans and having them adhered to by compliant patients. However, in the difficult days of my illness, I devised strategies for my survival, and I decided I could not afford to follow blindly the doctors' directions. During that intense struggle, I learned that not only was life a game, but so was the whole health-care industry.

Like any game, the health-care game is much easier to play if you know the rules. After years of hitting brick walls and making health-care decisions I didn't feel qualified to make, I discovered the rules by which the health-care industry operates. And I came up with my own set of rules to cope with the world of medicine.

Rule 1:
We Are Health-Care Consumers

People spend more time deciding where to go for dinner than they spend choosing their health-care providers. They put more time and effort into buying a television set than they put into choosing their doctors. They ask about the differences in quality among different television models and about available options, and they shop around for the best price. Once the decision has been made and the television comes home, if something goes wrong they return it and demand satisfaction.

That's how you need to approach health care. Investigate the options available in health-care providers: the doctors, the hospitals, and the pharmacies. Then check out those options. What are the differences? Which are the best choices for *you* and *your* family? If your choices don't meet your expectations, complain, demand satisfaction, or start a new search. This is the most important purchase you will ever make; your life depends on it!

Rule 2:
Work with Your Doctor
as a Team to Get the
Quality Care You Need

Most people feel that the doctor-patient relationship is adversarial, but it doesn't have to be. Find a doctor who will be your partner in getting the care you need. A doctor who is willing to work with you will explain all the available options and help you decide which course of treatment is best.

Find a good doctor who is willing to play on your team in the health-care game. Then start asking questions of your doctor, nurses, medical technicians, and your insurance company. If you don't understand the answers, ask more questions. If you don't like the answers, ask about different ways of doing things. If you're still not satisfied with the answers, *find a new doctor.*

Many people say they are afraid of going to the doctor. They don't want to go unless they're really sick. Most of the time they would rather take care of themselves than have to rely on someone else. You don't *have* to rely on a doctor. You need to find a doctor who will work with you as a team and help you decide on treatments that are right for *you!* Those who won't go to doctors because of fear are just tired of being treated as somehow less than the doctor's equal. So, find a doctor who wants to be a part of your team. That is your right as a health-care consumer.

Rule 3:
Medicine Is a Business

Medicine is the fastest-growing business in America, and all business practices apply, including negotiation. What, you may wonder, would you negotiate? How about fees? Medicare and insurance companies do it, and so can you! Doctors' fees are like prices for airline tickets: Rarely do all people pay the same price. Also like the airlines, doctors depend on repeat business, so *negotiate!*

Hospitals, laboratories, drug companies, and insurance companies, as well as other health-care providers, are in business to make a profit. These businesses spend enormous amounts of money on advertising, marketing, and promotion to convince doctors and patients to choose their services.

Health-care companies are very selective about who they allow to use their services. Hospitals and labs insist that patients have adequate health insurance coverage or adequate cash to pay their bills in full. But remember, you do have choices. *They* may want to do business with *you*, but do *you* want to do business with *them?*

Health Insurance Companies: A Preexisting Condition

Over 35 million people in the United States are not covered by any kind of health insurance. Health insurance companies strive to insure the healthy so they can collect premiums but not pay out on claims. As a result, those who have health problems are turned down or are given coverage only in exchange for astronomically high premiums.

In addition to those who have *no* health insurance, many are *underinsured*. If you currently have diabetes, a heart condition, or allergies, or if you're pregnant, a new health insurance policy may state that these "preexisting conditions" won't be covered for six months, for a year, or ever! That means you will remain uninsured for the very conditions for which you are most likely to require medical treatment. When looking into a new health insurance plan, you should scrutinize the "preexisting conditions" section very carefully.

Admittedly, health insurance itself has been changing. In the past, the more care provided, the more the health insurance companies paid out. Insurance companies capitalized on that fact. Their advertisements stated that they were "there when you need us." They were selling "peace of mind" as well as insurance. But now, we have health maintenance organizations (HMOs) and managed-care plans. In these instances the doctor receives a standardized payment per patient. Whether it takes one visit or four visits to cure the condition, the doctor earns the same amount.

The obvious intention of the health insurance companies has been to save money. HMOs make private agreements with drug companies to prescribe only those companies' products in exchange for guaranteed lower prices. This is not wrong; it is what all businesses have to do— *save* money as well as *make* money.

Hospitals and the Public Good

If you have any doubt that medicine is a business, consider why a hospital charges three dollars for a single aspirin. It's not because the hospital actually pays three dollars for each aspirin itself. The hospital wants to make money, even if that means charging up to ten times what an item actually costs.

With the approval of health insurance companies, hospitals use cost shifting to cover their unpaid bills. Cost shifting means that those with insurance are charged disproportionately high prices to make up for those who have no insurance and cannot pay their bills. I asked a health insurance executive why cost shifting would be allowed. He told me that the insurance companies did this "for the public good." I notice that I have never been consulted in making this decision, even though I'm the one who is directly affected each time I pay my medical bills!

Cost shifting will increase. HMOs work out special arrangements with doctors, labs, and hospitals to charge lower rates for their members. Medicare patients are charged at rates that are lower than the doctors' regular rates. These lower rates don't mean that these health-care providers are making less money, just that they're charging higher prices to those who are not on specialized insurance plans.

Attempts to rein in the costs of health care have resulted in the for-profit hospital. Corporate chain ownership has led to hospitals being run just like any other business: with an emphasis on profit and earnings. Even so, for-profit hospitals end up costing the public approximately 23 percent more than nonprofit hospitals cost. For years, the thinking was that the more hospital beds you had, the more money you were going to make. Then HMOs and managed-care came along. In order to cut costs, the lengths of hospital stays were shortened and outpatient surgeries were favored over inpatient procedures. What we have now is an overabundance of empty hospital beds.

For-profit hospitals have concerns that other hospitals don't. In addition to having to answer to insurance companies, patients, and doctors, they also have to consider the needs of their stockholders. Stockholders aren't really interested in the state of health care in general—all they want to do is make a profit on their investment.

Drug Companies and Popular Demand

Why would drug companies market a product that is virtually unnecessary? Because they're out to make a quick buck, too. Between 85 and 90 percent of adult incontinence, for instance, is treatable, but you certainly wouldn't realize that if you've watched the television commercials for adult diapers. Drug companies have told us that *this* is the way to deal with the situation. As a result, those who are too embarrassed to bring up the subject with their doctors will go to their local drugstores and, using manu-facturers' coupons, will buy adult diapers. The drug com-panies have done what all businesses try to do—create a demand for a product where no need yet exists.

Be as wary of advertisements for health-care products as you are of anything else you buy. Pay attention to tele-vision commercials. Currently there is a commercial pitch-ing formula for toddlers. I think this is an example of a company not having tested the market before introducing a new product. Parents I talked with told me their goal was to have their children eat regular food as soon as pos-sible, not keep them on special foods. Doctors have also told me that there is no good reason to buy this product and that you should save your money.

And what about weight-loss centers? Every January, like clockwork, two things happen: You have to start pay-ing your health insurance deductible all over again, and you see an onslaught of commercials for weight-loss cen-ters. Beware of their misleading claims. They promise unrealistic levels of weight loss and obscure the true cost of their programs. Find out if that $99 price to lose "all the weight you want" is the *complete* cost. Will you have to pay additional hundreds of dollars to use their food prod-ucts as well? These companies approach you as a cus-tomer, and you need to check them out. Most if not all of the "counselors" at these centers are salespeople. Their knowledge of nutrition and psychology is nonexistent. Ask about success rates—and people who come back over and over again don't count! You are looking for a long-term solution.

What can *you* do? Act like the health-care consumer you are. Question the purchases you make. Ask your doc-tor if this is the best way to solve your particular medical problem.

Be aware when buying over-the-counter (OTC) medications. Drug companies now give you a wide assortment
of OTC medications to choose from. Bayer, Tylenol,
Sudafed, and many other medicines can be bought to
"relieve symptoms" of various ailments. You can choose
from the "Cold and Flu Formula," the "Head Cold and
Fever Formula," and the "Nighttime Cold and Fever Formula." You can get them with aspirin, without aspirin, or
aspirin-free. It's important to note that the "aspirin-free"
and "without aspirin" formulas are not the same—one
uses acetaminophen and the other uses ibuprofen. But the
fact is that if you are not able to take aspirin, you probably should not be using ibuprofen, either. Read the pack-
aging carefully and make sure you know what you are
buying and whether it's going to work. Cold medications
that contain antihistamines, for example, won't work any
better than medications without them. Antihistamines relieve allergy symptoms, but they do nothing for the common cold.

Is using medication always the best choice? Sometimes
taking it easy and drinking lots of fluids would be better,
but of course it is not in the best interests of drug companies to promote this course of action. There's no money
in it. Illnesses can be categorized as viral and bacterial. If
you have a virus, antibiotics won't help. OTC medications
may lessen the symptoms, but basically the prescribed
course of action is usually to stay in bed for a few days.
So, don't take medicine (antibiotics) that won't work. Save
your money. Bacterial infections, on the other hand,
respond to antibiotics and can be cured when an appropriate course of treatment is followed.

Last year I was diagnosed with viral pneumonia. I did-
n't think it was serious since I was told to just stay home,
relax, and get better. I didn't. The viral pneumonia turned

into bacterial pneumonia. At this point my doctor explained how serious this condition was. It was contagious and unless the medicine she prescribed worked, I could wind up in the hospital. I thought the bacterial pneumonia was easier to get over since the antibiotics knocked it out.

Doctors

Doctors are not exempt from approaching medicine as a business. In fact, some doctors have a financial interest in medical labs. This is legal, although in some states—California, New York, and Connecticut, for instance—doctors are required to tell patients about any financial interest they have in a lab to which they make referrals. If your state has no such laws, the best way to protect *your* interest is to act like a consumer. Ask questions. Does your doctor have an ownership interest in a lab? Why is his lab better than an independent one?

When I was in the hospital having my daughter, my obstetrician asked an anesthesiologist to keep an eye on me because of my Hodgkin's disease. He also mentioned to the anesthesiologist that I would be having an operation one month later. For the two days I was in the hospital, my husband and I spoke with the anesthesiologist four times. (Most patients are lucky if they get to see their anesthesiologist once!) He gave us three business cards and asked us to request him when I came back in for my surgery. Under different circumstances I might have been impressed by this doctor's persistence, but at this time I wanted my well-being, not my future business, to be most important to the doctor.

One year later, I found myself using this doctor's services again. During his presurgery questioning, he asked me if I had read the three books he had written. Then he gave me the publisher's name and told me where I could buy them. He was only doing what any other business-person does—promoting his services and his products.

None of these practices is illegal or unethical. They are all simply standard operating procedure for good busi-ness. But be aware that medical products and services are marketed to you because you are a consumer, so you should choose whom you do business with very carefully.

Chapter 2

Finding the Best Doctor for You

When it comes to finding a good doctor, it's hard to know where to start. You have many choices: man or woman, old or young, traditional or holistic, general practitioner or specialist. Which physicians will your health insurance company authorize? Do you need a referral? If the doctor is not on your insurance plan, are you willing to pay the whole bill?

Take the time to decide what is important to you and your family before you start your search. Once you narrow down what you're looking for, you're ready to begin.

What Makes a Good Doctor?

Doctors and patients have different ideas about what makes a good doctor. Doctors will tell you a good doctor is knowledgeable, has the ability to diagnose and treat illness, and keeps current by reading the latest medical literature.

But patients take for granted that their doctors are well qualified and capable of practicing in their specialties. Patients want a doctor who will listen to them, take time with them, and not keep them waiting too long. What patients should *also* want is a doctor who will explain illnesses and medical procedures so they can understand what's happening to their bodies. And the smartest health-

11

care consumers want a doctor who will involve them in solving problems and will make wellness a team effort.

An August 15, 1990, *USA Today* poll asked patients why they liked their doctors. The top three reasons were

- "He's interested in me and not just my disease."
- "He has time for me and is willing to explain things and answer questions."
- "He takes my viewpoints and questions seriously."

As in dealing with practitioners of any other occupation, you should never assume that all doctors are good. Of course, that doesn't mean you can't find a good doctor. It just means you have to consider every doctor carefully. If you read the newspaper you get used to stories about doctors with questionable track records. There *are* doctors who've been sued for malpractice many times and even had their licenses revoked, but it's possible to avoid those. Get referrals and check credentials. That is your right as a health care consumer, and your obligation to yourself and your family.

Requesting Referrals

The best way to find a new doctor is to ask everyone you know. How do they like their doctor? Most important, ask whether they would recommend their doctor to you.

Family, Friends, Neighbors, and Coworkers

The most popular way of finding a new doctor is by talking to family and friends, neighbors and coworkers.

When asking those around you to recommend a doctor, find out *why* they like him. Maybe your friend's doctor is outgoing, constantly asking questions about her lifestyle and making suggestions on how to improve her general well-being. Every appointment she has turns into a gab-fest, and she always leaves the doctor's office with suggestions for how to enhance her life. This may be fine for her, but maybe you would prefer someone who'll just listen to your concerns, come up with a diagnosis, and get you on your way. Everyone has different needs in the doctor-patient relationship. Your brother's needs ("He gets me in and out of the office fast, he doesn't ask personal questions, and his office is across the street from my job") may not be the same as yours. In fact, you may want to avoid his doctor.

Your Current Doctor, Nurse, and Pharmacist

Of course, doctors believe that the best way to find a new doctor is to get a referral from a current doctor or nurse or from the pharmacist at your drugstore. I usually ask one of my doctors to recommend a new doctor for me. The advantage in this is that my doctor knows my personality and that of the doctor he's referring me to. This approach usually provides me with a good match. If you are comfortable with this strategy, go to a health-care provider you trust and ask her whom she would consider if she were looking for a doctor for her family. If you already have the names of some doctors, ask what she thinks of your candidates. No doctor, nurse, or pharmacist will tell you that a particular doctor is bad, but they might indicate whether one would suit you better than another.

Call hospitals in your area and ask to speak with a charge nurse. If you're looking for a surgeon, ask for the charge nurse on the surgery floor; if you're looking for a pediatrician, ask for the charge nurse on the pediatrics floor. Ask the nurse for her recommendation. Nurses know which doctors are good and which ones aren't. But don't mention any doctors' names or ask what the nurse thinks of particular doctors. This is an extremely awkward situation for any hospital employee. You're more likely to get a good referral if you just ask the nurse to name some names. Ask who *she* would go to if she were looking for a new doctor.

Referral Services

Doctor-referral services advertise frequently on radio and television. They are also listed in the yellow pages. But you should be aware that physicians pay a fee to be listed with a referral service, so these names are not given out just for the public good. However, you will be able to find out where the doctor went to school, if she is board certified, how long she's been practicing, where her office is, and what her office hours are.

Hospitals have their own referral services—but, of course, they will refer you only to doctors who practice at that hospital.

Health Insurance Plans

Many insurance policies restrict you to doctors associated with their plan. If you are enrolled in one of these plans, you'll be choosing a doctor from a limited, pre-approved list. Keep in mind that a doctor who is part of a health insurance plan has gone through no screening process. He has simply filled out an application and agreed to charge the prices authorized by the insurance company.

So, before you choose from that short list, you will still need to check out thoroughly every doctor you're considering.

While you are doing all this research, you may notice that one doctor's name gets mentioned over and over. That's a good sign. Along with the list of reasons that others think he's a great doctor, it could even be the deciding factor.

One very important "don't"—Never choose a doctor from the Yellow Pages! When I mention this in my seminars, I notice there are two groups of people laughing: those who can't believe anyone would ever look for a doctor in the yellow pages, and those who have done it.

> *One very important "don't"—Never choose a doctor from the* **Yellow Pages!**

Checking Credentials

As in any other business, people can say anything they want about their background and experience; it doesn't mean that it's true. Once you have the names of doctors who interest you, check out their credentials.

American Medical Association

Contact the American Medical Association 312-464-5199; 515 North State Street, Chicago, Ill. 60610. If you are prepared to be put on hold, deal with their personnel, and have their voicemail system hang up on you, you can get some important information on doctors. They will be able to tell you if the doctor is licensed to practice medicine in your state. They will also be able to tell you when she received her license, where she went to school, and whether she is licensed in other states. But you should know that not all doctors are members of this association. The American Medical Association has a dues-paying membership. I suggest that you contact this group by mail. You can also receive this information from your state medical association.

Official ABMS Directory Of Board-Certified Medical Specialists

This multivolume book can be found at your public library (Reed Reference Publishing Co., 121 Chanlon Road, New Providence, N.J. 07974). It contains basic information: where the doctor is licensed to practice, how long she has practiced, where she went to school, and what her medical specialty is. In addition to traditional specialists, this book also covers general practitioners and family physicians.

American Board of Medical Specialty

The American Board of Medical Specialty (800-776-2378; 47 Perimeter Center East, Suite 500, Atlanta, Ga. 30346) will tell you whether a doctor is board certified. "Board certified" means that a doctor has taken additional classes in his specialty, has practiced in that specialty for a number of years, and has passed the required tests.

Watch out for the phrase "board eligible." A doctor who is board eligible has taken the additional classes necessary for board certification but has not taken or passed the required tests.

Ask your doctor if he is board certified. If he says he is board eligible, you may want to ask why he hasn't completed certification. If a doctor is young and has just begun practicing, he may need to work for a couple of years before he is able to take these tests. Most group practices will not allow a doctor to remain with the practice if he is not able to pass the tests and become board certified.

State Medical Licensing Board

Your local state medical licensing board will be able to tell you when a doctor was first licensed, the status of his license, and the standing of the doctor with the board. Ask if the doctor has been subject to misconduct charges or disciplinary actions.

Questionable Doctors

Check the reference section of your public library for the book *Questionable Doctors* (Public Citizen Health Research Group, Dept. QD2, 2000 P Street NW, No. 700, Washington, D.C. 20036). It lists doctors who've been disciplined by state or federal agencies for malpractice or misconduct. It is revised annually.

National Practitioners Data Bank

There is a tremendous need for one source where patients can access all the information they need to research doctors. Currently, such a source does not exist. It is not even possible to find out whether a doctor has practiced in other states, if he doesn't want anyone to know.

A Harvard University malpractice study showed that doctors kill more than 75,000 Americans every year through medical negligence. That's more than all accidental deaths in the United States annually.[1]

---

[1] Paul C. Weiler, Howard H. Hiatt, Joseph P. Newhouse, William G. Johnson, Troyen A. Brennan, and Lucian L. Leape, 1993, *A Measure of Malpractice; Medical Injury, Malpractice Litigation, and Patient Compensation,* Cambridge, Mass., Harvard University Press.

Even if a doctor has been sued countless times and has moved from one state to another to avoid prosecution, you won't be able to find this out. Most hospitals will reprimand a doctor "unofficially," barring him from practicing at that hospital but taking no disciplinary action that might restrict him from working elsewhere. This is an example of "sundowning," when inept doctors are pushed out of one state with no provisions for alerting hospitals or patients in the state where they'll practice next.

The Health Care Quality Improvement Act of 1986 established a data bank that the U.S. Department of Health and Human Services has been compiling since September 1990, including incompetent or frequently sued doctors, dentists, nurses, and other health professionals. Not surprisingly, the American Medical Association resists giving the public any access to this data bank.

The original intent of establishing the National Practitioner Data Bank was to force hospitals, licensing boards, HMOs, and other medical groups to guard against employing incompetent health practitioners. It's hard to make an argument that patients and consumers should not have access to this information as well.

When a woman I know became pregnant, she consulted her health insurance plan's list of doctors and chose one. Unfortunately, the doctor-patient relationship did not turn out to be what she wanted or needed. She felt that the doctor was insensitive, uncaring, and incompetent.

My client then did what all patients should do when they come across a doctor who they believe delivers substandard care. She filed a complaint with her health insurance company, the doctors' group where the doctor practiced, the hospital where the doctor had privileges to practice, the local medical association, the medical board of the state where she lives, and the American College of Obstetricians and Gynecologists.

Her initial complaint was lodged in January 1994. Six months later, in July 1994, I contacted all the institutions named above to see what had been done.

The insurance company was still referring patients to this doctor, stating that no complaints had been made against her. When I mentioned I was following up on a complaint that had been submitted in January, the company's spokesperson admitted that several patients had lodged complaints but that she didn't know what they were in reference to or if they were true. The insurance company continues to recommend the doctor.

The head of the doctors' group had already contacted my client by letter and suggested she be "real sure of your facts" before she said anything else about the doctor or they would sue her for libel.

A written reply from the head of the OB-GYN department at the hospital where this doctor practiced stated, "The hospital has no authority or judgment over the medical care rendered outside the confines of the hospital." The department head told me that, unless a doctor committed malpractice on the hospital premises, there was nothing the department could do. Because of the fear of a lawsuit, it is extremely unusual for any hospital to withdraw a doctor's privileges.

The state medical board informed me that no disciplinary actions had been taken against this doctor, but they refused to tell me if any complaints had been lodged. It was, they said, none of my business. That's funny, I thought—I'd say that the general public is *exactly* whose business it was.

You may be wondering whose rights the medical community is concerned about, the patient's or the doctor's. Even the courts have entered the struggle. In 1993, California Superior Court Judge Ronald Robie ruled that physicians' privacy rights outweigh the public's interest in finding out about complaints that have been filed against doctors. This judge feels that if a doctor is potentially dangerous to patients, the state should merely speed up the investigative process.

This is not a hopeless situation. Let your doctors and members of congress know that the National Practitioners Data Bank should be accessible to doctors and consumers alike. Better health care serves everyone's best interests.

A Patient's Right to Choose

Everyone would like to be able to choose the best doctors and methods of medical treatment, but this is no longer possible. With more health insurance companies relying on managed-care, our options are becoming limited. The limiting factor is money. What treatments are cost effective? Which treatments are *worth* that cost?

As consumers, we must be realistic. Not all medical problems or illnesses can be cured. Throwing money at those problems isn't always the answer. Some states have already come to that realization. The State of Oregon has devised a health plan that provides care to the state's low-income disabled and elderly residents (as a supplement to Medicare). This health plan is centered around a prioritized list of health services, which includes some 745 medical conditions. The items on the list are ordered by how well these conditions respond to medical intervention and by the cost involved in that care.

Oregon's health plan is being watched carefully by others to see if it is feasible to implement a similar plan in their own state. The main concern seems to be that there is no room for special considerations. Everything is dealt with in a cut-and-dried manner.

HMOs and managed-care organizations are very interested in this concept. They are now limiting access to specialists, and in the future they may refuse treatment for specific conditions under certain circumstances. As a consumer it is important for you to stand up for your needs. Learn what your options are and what kind of treatment is appropriate—then *fight* for it.

What to Do When You Need a Specialist

If your doctor is a member of a managed-care health insurance plan, you may find that she is extremely reluctant to have you see a specialist. It could be that your doctor feels she can handle the problem herself, but chances are that her managed-care plan operates with a "shared risk pool." In most managed-care plans, a pool of money is set aside to be used for testing and visits to specialists for patients. If this pool of money is not used up by the end of the term, the doctor gets to keep it for herself. This could become a conflict of interest; the best interests of the patient are different from those of the doctor.

If your doctor has been treating a medical problem for a couple of weeks and nothing seems to be working, be assertive. Tell her you think it's time you saw a specialist and ask directly which one she suggests. Make sure that the specialist your doctor recommends is part of your health-care plan so that your visits will be covered.

If you are not on a managed-care plan, it is still a good idea to have a general practitioner or primary care physician watching over your health care and suggesting specialists as needed. If you are only going to a specialist when you have a problem with your health, you may not receive the complete care you need. If you go to an OB-GYN, she will be looking for problems specifically dealing with gynecology. Other problems may be overlooked because they are not within her specialty.

General practitioners and primary care physicians have a basic knowledge of many diseases. They have had over three years of training encompassing a variety of medical conditions. This does *not* mean that they should be treating heart-failure or cancer patients; primary care physicians do not have the extensive knowledge of these diseases that specialists do. They may not know of the newest research or treatment techniques available. For that you need a specialist.

What to Do When Your Doctor Leaves a Group Practice

Another problem patients face is what to do when their doctor leaves a group practice or is no longer covered on their health insurance plan.

More and more, health insurance plans are choosing doctors on the basis of their ability to run an inexpensive practice. Managed-care plans, striving to be the most cost-effective, well-managed programs possible, often drop doctors who order more expensive tests than their colleagues. The *Wall Street Journal* found that Prudential and Aetna Insurance in Houston had terminated dozens of physicians for that reason. The *Wall Street Journal* reported Pilgrim Health Care in Boston's intention to end its ten-year affiliation with New England Medical Center, a big teaching and research hospital, effective February 1995.[2] The termination included its 300 doctors. The reason for these terminations was simply a matter of money. Cheaper health care was available elsewhere.

---

[2]*Wall Street Journal,* December 30, 1993, p. 1.

If your doctor's office is dropped from your health insurance plan in favor of other doctors, you still have the option of continuing to see your doctor, but at increased cost. This may be necessary if you are being treated for an ongoing condition. Under these circumstances, let your doctor know about your situation and see if you can negotiate fees that you can reasonably handle.

Some doctors' employment contracts prevent them from taking patients with them if they leave one group practice to join another. Health professionals state that these clauses interfere with patients' rights to be treated by doctors with whom they've had an extensive relationship. The quality of patients' health care is also an issue here, because new doctors won't be as familiar with these patients' medical histories.

Courts are beginning to understand these problems and are refusing to enforce contracts that penalize doctors for taking patients with them when they leave a practice. In 1992, a Florida court ruled that such contracts interfere with the patient's right to choose.

Sometimes you have to be creative to keep a doctor you like. When I was pregnant and had already been diagnosed with cancer, my husband's company changed health insurance plans. This was a very scary time for me. I trusted my oncologist and we had decided on a treatment plan. I was satisfied with the present situation and was not willing to change. When we received the list of doctors on our new plan, I showed it to my oncologist and asked him to recommend an internist who was associated with the plan. When I went to see the internist, I told him that the oncologist had referred me to him and asked for an ongoing referral to the oncologist. It worked. I was able to continue seeing the doctor of my choice. There is usually a way to get what you want from your

health-care providers. Approach the situation as a consumer. Do what you *need* to do to get the quality care you
want!

You may not have the luxury of enough time to check
out a new doctor. In that case, if you are happy with the
care you receive from your current doctor, rely on his
opinion. If you are in the hospital, ask the nurses.

I was five months pregnant when the internist sus-
pected I had cancer. I had found a lump in my neck and
went to the doctor expecting to be reassured that it was
nothing serious. Instead, the doctor gave me an emotion-
less diagnosis of malignant melanoma. After sending me
down the hall to get X rays taken, he made an appointment for me to see an ear, nose, and throat doctor an hour
later for a needle biopsy. The next morning my husband
and I were talking with an oncologist about my options.
That evening I was in the hospital for an outpatient biopsy
procedure. Less than twenty-four hours after that I had a
confirmed diagnosis of Hodgkin's disease.

Throughout this process of being sent from one doctor to another and having one diagnostic test after another,
I started feeling that everything was out of my control. But
I didn't leave the choice of doctors to chance. I stayed in
close contact with my obstetrician. In addition to making
sure that the medical procedures wouldn't adversely affect
my baby, I discussed with him the other specialists necessary for my treatment. Because of this, I was consistently
passed along to the best doctor in any given specialty.
When I was in the hospital for the biopsy, I asked the
surgery nurse what she thought of the surgeon. She showed
me a very faint scar on her arm and told me the same doctor had operated on her a month before and had done a
great job.

Most doctors are highly educated, know their specialty, and want to make people feel better. Your job is to search out those doctors and work together with them to get yourself the health care that you deserve.

Chapter 3

The Doctor–Health-Care Consumer Team

The "Get-Acquainted" Appointment

Now that you've done your research and found a good doctor, call the office and make a "get-acquainted" appointment. Notice how quickly the phone is answered and how soon you can be scheduled for an appointment. The get-acquainted appointment is your chance to interview the doctor. Most doctors will not charge for this visit.

Some questions you will want to ask the doctor are: How do I reach you? What is the best time to call? How long does it take for you to respond to your messages? Who fills in for you when you're not available? If this doctor is a specialist, you will want to make sure that the doctor who fills in for him is a specialist as well.

What are the doctor's office hours? Early? Late? Including Saturdays? Doctors are beginning to realize that many patients are unable to make it to the office between nine and five Monday through Friday and are now extending their office hours. If your doctor has not yet done this, ask if he is considering doing it in the future.

Find out if the doctor makes house calls. Although many people think this practice stopped in the days of the horse and carriage, some doctors have started it up again. It's now becoming prevalent with elderly patients.

The doctor's answers will let you know how you will be treated as a patient in his practice. If you are kept waiting for a long period of time, or the doctor doesn't pay attention to your questions, perhaps he is not the right doctor for you. How much time did the doctor set aside for your appointment? If he is trying to end it before you have a chance to get answers to all your questions, he will probably not give you sufficient time when you come in sick.

Let the doctor know that you are looking for a *team* relationship and not just someone to dictate to you. Ask him if he is comfortable with this kind of arrangement. Make sure that the doctor's views on health care mesh with your own. Does he depend on X rays as a diagnostic tool? Many doctors are concerned about excess exposure to radiation, believing that there is a correlation between radiation doses and cancer risk.[1] They prefer to limit the number of X rays taken. Does he prescribe antibiotics indiscriminately? Doctors are beginning to realize that overprescribing antibiotics lessens their impact. Be sure that the doctor realizes that your goal is the same as his, keeping you healthy.

In my seminars, I've had many people complain that doctors call patients by their first names, while the doctors insist on being called "Doctor." This issue seems to be of more concern to older patients whose doctors are much younger than they are. Discuss this with the doctor. If you would prefer that he call you by your last name, let him know that. On the other hand, you might not mind having him call you by your first name, but you want to refer to him in the same way. Let your doctor know that this would make you feel more equal in your relationship.

---

[1]Peter Radetsky, "The Mad-As-Hell Scientist," *Longevity*, February 1995, p. 62.

I had always felt comfortable calling my doctors "Doctor," and I didn't mind if they called me by my first name. It wasn't until I began treatment with my oncologist that I encountered another approach. I had called the doctor's office in the afternoon with a concern I had. Later that night, around nine o'clock, the phone rang. When I answered the phone, "Bob" told me he was returning my call from earlier in the day. It took a while before I realized that Bob was my oncologist!

Bring All Your Medications with You

It is extremely important that your doctor knows what drugs you are taking. All medications have some potential side effects, and the doctor may need to know if symptoms you are having could be caused by drugs you are taking. Put all your medications, prescription and over-the-counter, in a bag and bring them with you. In addition to learning what drugs you are taking and in what dosage, your doctor will need to know how often and for how long you've been taking them.

With the get-acquainted appointment, your goal is to see if you can work as a team with this doctor. Do your styles mesh?

Beware of the doctor who won't meet with you for the first time with your clothes on!

Beware of the doctor who won't meet with you for the first time with your clothes on!

Make Yourself Known to the Doctor's Staff

Some people bypass the doctor's staff as often as possible, choosing to speak only with the doctor. This is a big mistake. The most important reason to get to know the doctor's staff is that many doctors have extensive practices and it is hard for them to remember all of their patients.

You will get better care if the office staff knows who you are. That way, they will have a greater interest in your well-being.

Introduce yourself to the nurses, the secretaries, and the rest of the office staff. When calling the office for an appointment or information, identify yourself and ask to whom you are speaking. It's harder for someone to give you a hard time when they know that they're not anonymous.

The Doctor's Appointment

Since you will be working with your doctor as a team, it is important that you take an active part in this relationship. Come to your appointments well prepared; this practice will help you receive the best possible care.

Bring a List of Questions with You

Going to the doctor can be a stressful experience. You won't always remember everything you want to discuss, so always bring a list of questions with you. At the top of the list should be the item that is bothering you the most. Most people wait until the end of the doctor's appointment before mentioning why they are really there, and it is said that doctors listen for only about eighteen seconds before they interrupt the patient's statement of concerns. If both these assertions are true, then doctors rarely get a chance to hear about the real problem. Tell your doctor that you want her to listen to *all* your concerns before she starts telling you what's wrong. This should ensure that the doctor will be concentrating on what you're saying.

Don't be afraid to question your doctor. Are there different approaches to recovery? You know your lifestyle better than she does. Tell her what you will be able to do and help your doctor work out the best plan of attack. For instance, instead of taking medicine three or four times a day, is there a different drug that can be taken once a day? When my daughter had a sinus infection her pediatrician prescribed an antibiotic that needed to be taken every six hours. My child was in school at the time and I wasn't sure how to do this. I explained my dilemma to the doctor and she changed the prescription to a drug to be taken once a day. Similar problems have come up at other times with my daughter. Once a liquid antibiotic that needed to be refrigerated was prescribed. We were about to go on vacation, so I asked if it was possible to find a chewable pill instead.

Another reason to question a plan of treatment is when it's just not working. If you're supposed to be better in three days and you're getting worse, ask the doctor what else you should try.

When a test is scheduled, ask what it's for, what the side effects are, and whether there are other options. Ask the doctor what she expects the test results to reveal and what will be the next step after that. If your doctor recommends surgery, ask if alternative treatments are available. How long will the convalescence be? Will the surgeon do the surgery herself or have a resident do it? Will the surgery be performed on an inpatient or outpatient basis? Will you need someone to care for you once you get home? How many times has the doctor performed this procedure? It is important that the doctor have had experience with this specific procedure. For safety, the surgeon should have done a minimum of forty to fifty of the same surgeries you are considering, yearly. You do not want to be practice for the doctor.

Don't be afraid to interrupt and have your doctor explain everything clearly. Your doctor may want to "give orders," but if you do not understand or are not willing to comply with those orders, you will not get better.

If you don't know what questions to ask, say, "If you were me, what would you ask?" Health-care consumers know that working as a team to find a plan that will work for you will ensure that you receive better-quality health care.

The "Difficult" Patient

Some people have told me that they can't imagine questioning a doctor. They don't want the doctor, or his staff, to see them as a difficult patient. I have never seen myself as a difficult patient. I am simply standing up for the care I need. I am a health-care consumer. The questions I raise and the solutions I seek are for the express purpose of seeing that my family and I receive the quality health care we require.

It is up to *you* to question the care you receive. If you don't ask questions and insist on quality care for yourself and your loved ones, no one else will.

Get Answers to Your Questions

Asking questions is not enough. You have to make sure that you are getting answers to those questions. Answers such as "Got me!", "Gee, that's interesting!", or "I've never seen that before!" are not what you're looking for. Ask what you should do. If the doctor doesn't know what to suggest, ask if she will be researching it or referring you to another doctor.

Be careful of the doctor who is always saying, "Let's wait and see." Most of the people in my seminars don't go to the doctor unless they feel something is truly wrong.

They've already waited as long as they can. Tell your doctor you don't want to put off treatment any longer than you already have.

If You Don't Understand, Ask for a Better Explanation

Don't be embarrassed if you don't understand "doctor speak." It's your doctor who should be embarrassed for resorting to high-tech talk. Tell the doctor that you don't understand what he's saying and that you need a clearer or simpler explanation. When you think you understand your doctor's instructions, repeat them to make sure.

Bring a Friend or Family Member with You to Your Appointment

If you don't feel comfortable asking your doctor questions, bring a family member or close friend with you to listen to the doctor and ask questions that you may not think of. This is particularly important if you have a serious illness. When you are not feeling well, you may not be able to concentrate on what the doctor is telling you.

When I was first diagnosed with cancer, my husband came with me to my doctor appointments. We often heard what the doctor said differently and even had to call the office to clarify what had been said. Another advantage of having someone there with you is that they can ask questions you don't want to ask. I never asked if I was going to die, though it was something I had thought about; my husband asked that question. I let my doctor know that it was important for him to talk to my husband. If my husband called with questions or wanted to know any information on my case, he was to be told. There is a confidentiality agreement called the doctor-patient privilege, but if you want someone else to be able to get the same information from your doctor that you would, tell your doctor that you want them to have that kind of access.

Before You Leave the Doctor's Office

Before you leave your doctor's office, make sure you understand the recommended treatment. Do you have a cold, or the flu, or strep throat? Ask the doctor if you are contagious. Will he prescribe medicine? Do you need complete bed rest, or can you go to work as usual?

What are the instructions for taking the medicine? Should you stop taking other drugs you are currently taking? Can you still go to the gym to work out or should you wait for a couple of days? When will you start feeling better? Are you supposed to come back to be rechecked? Can you just call the office to let them know that you are better?

Whenever you are meeting with your doctor or talking with him on the phone, remember you are working together as a team. When he suggests a treatment or procedure, ask him why he feels that is the best way to handle the problem. If you don't agree, let him know why. If you've heard or read something about your condition, ask the doctor what he thinks about it. Together you will be able to make sure that you are getting the health care you need.

Sources of Information on Health-Care Issues

Doctors keep up to date on health-care issues by reading medical journals and talking with other health-care professionals. The health-care consumer needs to keep up to date on these issues as well.

The Media: Television, Newspapers, Magazines, and Radio

Watch the nightly news and you will hear that the flu season is here and it's time to get a flu shot. Read the morning newspaper and you will learn about a new treatment for migraine headaches. Go to the newsstand and scan the current magazine covers. You will see articles on how taking vitamins prevents cancer, how to cope with back pain, how to eliminate the stress in your life, or how to tell if you're depressed. Listen to a radio talk show and you will hear discussions on various illnesses, treatments, and new discoveries.

Did you know that snoring has been linked to high blood pressure, heart attacks, and strokes? That men whose mothers took the drug DES when pregnant have a higher rate of depression and alcoholism? You can learn a lot about medicine by listening, reading, and watching various forms of media. When something about your condition or lifestyle or chronic illnesses catches your attention, write it down, or cut out the article and mention it to your doctor the next time you see him. Ask if he's heard about it and find out what he thinks.

Computer Databases and Bulletin Boards

The computer age has given doctors greater access to information that will help them with their diagnostic skills. There are computer programs like Help, QMR, and Apache that help doctors evaluate patient care. These computer programs are not meant to replace doctors, just to help them out.

But computers are also a help to the health-care consumer. CompuServe, America Online, Prodigy, and Delphi are just a few of the on-line computer services with databases, bulletin boards, and health forums that can provide you with information you wouldn't be able to find elsewhere. The United Cerebral Palsy Association and the National Multiple Sclerosis Society are represented on America Online. Prodigy has health-care forums dealing with colitis and multiple sclerosis. You can also tap into the database "Homework Helper," where you can look up articles on health-care concerns in various magazines and periodicals, including the *Los Angeles Times, USA Today, Psychology Today,* and many more. You can even buy reasonably priced computer software programs that will help you diagnose your problems, teach you first aid, and keep records of your medical care.

When using both computer on-line systems and software programs, it is very important to remember that you should not try to become your own doctor. The information that is available is not being offered *just* for the public good. There may be ulterior motives at work. Discuss the information that you find with your doctor. She does have substantial knowledge and experience that you don't have and that computer programs can't give you.

Medical Libraries and Public Libraries

Most, if not all, hospitals have medical libraries that doctors, nurses, and other medical professionals use to research medical issues. These libraries can be used by the general public as well, but you may find the writing in medical books and journals to be extremely technical and difficult to understand.

Public libraries are great resources for finding information you may need. The librarian can direct you to specific books or tell you about groups in your community that will have answers to your questions. In addition to looking up medical terms and having them explained clearly, you will also be able to locate newspaper and magazine articles written on many medical topics. Your public library may also have a computer database called Infotrak that you could find useful. It's easy to use even if you have no prior computer experience.

Health Resource Centers

More and more people want to know how they can improve their health and the health of their families. Hospitals have responded to this interest by opening health resource centers, which can be an endless source of helpful information. These centers have pamphlets available on many medical conditions, as well as general information on keeping yourself healthy. You can find books on all kinds of subjects at these centers as well, including pregnancy, children's health, and low-fat cooking. You may also be able to find information on alternative medical practices, such as "natural" healing with herbs, biofeedback, and homeopathic remedies.

Some centers offer health screenings and information on where you can rent infant car seats or "baby beepers." Pagers or beepers were once used primarily by busy professionals who couldn't afford to be away from the phone; now this concept works well for fathers-to-be who don't want to miss the "big moment."

These centers can also tell you about support groups that help participants deal with specific medical concerns like how to be a caregiver, how to cope with the emotional stress of cancer, or how to handle the death of a loved one.

Medical Associations: Heart, Cancer, Diabetes . . .

You can always get current health-care information from your local medical associations. They will be able to send you information on specific subjects, including treatment plans that are currently approved for use by doctors. They will have the most up-to-date information on recent advances as well as the names of specialists in your area. They can also put you in touch with patient groups for counseling.

It's important for you to remember that as a health-care consumer, you are never alone in your search to get the best medical information and care. Discuss what you find out with your doctor. Treatments, procedures, and developments you read about might not pertain to your particular situation, but don't be afraid to mention them to your doctor. It's possible that your doctor may not have discussed these alternatives with you because he didn't think you would be interested. Perhaps he felt they wouldn't work in your situation, or maybe he didn't know enough about them.

What to Do When
Your Doctor Doesn't Know
What's Wrong

The doctor–health-care consumer relationship is based on trust and confidence. You trust that your doctor will always do what is best for you, and you have confidence that he will *know* what is best for you. Is that confidence well placed? An article in the August 1993 issue of *McCall's* magazine asserted that not all doctors are practicing up-to-date medicine.[2] Physicians seemed to fall short in three ways:

1. Underusing new and effective treatments
2. Continuing to use certain older therapies that have been shown to be ineffective or even harmful
3. Not knowing the latest diagnostic information

There is nothing wrong with a doctor who doesn't have all the answers. The question becomes what does your doctor do when he *knows* he doesn't.

Just as I was finishing chemotherapy treatment in 1991, I started getting persistent, severe pain in my back and legs. My oncologist didn't know the cause. I was admitted to the hospital for tests. When the tests came back inconclusive, specialists were called in. One and a half weeks later, when a rash broke out all over my body, I was diagnosed with shingles. The difficulty in diagnosing my case came from the fact that shingles usually *begins* with a rash. I didn't get the rash until several days later.

Illness and disease do not always match the descriptions in the medical textbooks. Will your doctor take the time and make the effort necessary to come up with a diagnosis? Does he keep up with current medical literature? If he doesn't know what to do, will he put you in touch with the specialists who do?

What should you do if you've been *mis*diagnosed? If the treatment prescribed doesn't work and the condition

---

[2]Leslie Laurence, "Three Mistakes Even Good Doctors Make," *McCall's,* August 1993.

persists, question the original diagnosis. Ask your doctor to refer you to a specialist. If a specialist can't help, consider going to a medical center.

If your doctor is always telling you, "I don't know" or "Let's just wait and see," it may be time to *find a new doctor.* Remember, that is your right as a health-care consumer.

Chapter 4

Finding a New and Better Doctor

You may have a doctor you think is wonderful and swear that you'll never change. I hope that's true. But it's not very likely. At some point in your health care, because of changes in your health insurance plan or some lifestyle change, you'll need to think about making a change.

It is imperative that you have a good relationship with your doctor. People who feel that their doctors don't communicate well with them are less likely to follow their doctors' instructions and less likely to report that their condition improved.[1] If you don't have a good relationship with your doctor, *change doctors.*

Twelve Reasons to Change Doctors

You Receive "Poor-Quality" Care

If you have concerns about the quality of care you are receiving from your doctor, it may be time to find a new one. If you have a chronic problem that you've discussed with your doctor many times, but you're still not better and the doctor isn't sure why—it's time to *find a new doctor.*

---

[1]"How Is Your Doctor Treating You?" *Consumer Reports,* February 1995, pp. 81–87.

If your doctor keeps ordering new tests to find out what's wrong but never finds an answer—it's time to *find a new doctor.*

First, talk to your doctor about your concerns. Does he think you should see a specialist? If you are seeing a specialist, perhaps you're seeing the wrong kind. Does the specialist know what's wrong? If he wants to do more tests, ask what he expects to learn from the results. One woman I know went to the doctor with a bad case of bronchitis. She was given medicine and told to come back if she wasn't better in two weeks. Two weeks later, still sick, she went back to the doctor. He told her he wanted to perform five separate tests and procedures. When she asked what he expected to find out from the results, he said, "Not much." The fact was that he ordered the tests because he thought that's what she wanted done.

Sometimes when we do not get well as fast as we want to, we blame it on poor-quality care. Doctors need to make sure that patients understand what to expect. When a doctor says, "You'll feel better in two weeks," find out whether he means "back to normal" or just "not coughing and sneezing all the time."

When I was undergoing radiation therapy, the doctor said he saw no reason why I wouldn't be able to work throughout the five weeks of treatment. From the first day of my treatment, I could barely get out of bed in the morning. I couldn't understand why I didn't have the energy to go back to work. In talking to other patients, however, I found that this was a pretty normal reaction. The other radiation patients had also been told by their doctors that they would be able to carry on with their lives as usual.

In this case I had not been expecting something unrealistic; rather, I had not been told how things were actually going to be. A doctor will often withhold the truth intentionally on the assumption that if he tells you what is *really* going to happen, your imagination will make it even worse. But a patient has the right to know exactly what to expect in his treatment. Talk to your doctor; tell him you want to know what to expect, realistically. If your doctor insists that he has it "under control" or that you have "nothing to worry about" when your experience tells you otherwise, *find a new doctor.* That is your right as a health-care consumer!

You may have found that it takes a long time for your doctor to figure out what's wrong with you and even longer to decide how to fix it. You've considered changing doctors but have been with this one forever and don't want to hurt his feelings. When it comes to your health, however, the only thing you should be concerned with is the care you are receiving. *Find yourself a new doctor* and keep the old one as a friend. If your car mechanic was a nice guy but he never fixed your car, you'd change mechanics, wouldn't you?

Most patients worry when their doctor's response to the question of what's wrong with them is "I don't know." This is not a bad answer, but if you have a good doctor, he'll go on to tell you what he's going to do to find out. When I was pregnant and diagnosed with Hodgkin's disease, I kept hearing how unusual my situation was. When it came to deciding if I should start treatment immediately or wait until my baby was born, my oncologist said he wasn't sure. But he told me immediately that he had a couple of friends who worked at Stanford University Hospital, where the cure for Hodgkin's was found. He called them and discussed the situation. My doctor may not have known what to do right away, but he sure knew where to go to find out.

You Have a "Poor Relationship" with Your Doctor

A good doctor-patient relationship is crucial to the health-care consumer. You have to feel comfortable enough to discuss anything, even embarrassing issues, with your doctor in order to receive the care you need. If this is not possible, *find a new doctor.*

Maybe you have a great relationship with your doctor, but you still hate going. When I was just out of college, I had a terrific doctor, but I still hated going to his office. Eventually I realized that this was because the nurse always wanted to weigh me, even when there was no reason to. I found myself putting off going to the doctor even when I should have gone because I didn't want a nurse to tell me that I should lose weight. One day, the nurse told me to get on the scale and I said, "Not today. If the doctor needs that information, I'll discuss it with him." When the doctor came into the examining room, I heard the nurse tell him I was a difficult patient. I may have been, but I was never weighed again there except when necessary.

Once I stood up for myself, the problem was solved. If you don't like how you're being treated at the doctor's office, see if you can change the situation. Not only are you a patient, you are also a *customer!*

Your Doctor Displays a Lack of Interest

When you're talking to your doctor, telling her of your concerns or describing the symptoms you've been having, does her mind seem to be somewhere else? When you ask questions, does she ignore them and then ask you questions of her own? This behavior could be a sign of a lack of interest in your problems or of a busy doctor who's still thinking about the patient she just left. Neither situation spells quality care for you.

Doctors working in managed-care networks often have to treat too many patients in a single day. Instead of being able to spend fifteen to twenty minutes with each patient, they may find themselves restricted to five minutes each, with no time in between.

Talk to your doctor about your concerns. Ask if she has time to see you or if she would prefer you find another doctor. Often, when confronted, the doctor will admit she was unaware that she was being inattentive. After your discussion, you may find her taking a special interest in your needs.

Your Doctor Exhibits Rude Behavior

"Bedside manner" is not a required course in medical school, and many doctors won't win a congeniality award, but this does not mean they have the right to be rude. More and more patients expect the relationship with their doctor to be one of equals. If your doctor does not feel comfortable with this arrangement or persists in being condescending or rude to you, *change doctors.*

Of course, what you perceive as rude may be simply a lack of social skills. When my husband and I first moved to Portland, Oregon, we were referred to an "excellent internist," but we were told that this doctor had absolutely *no* bedside manner; he was an excellent diagnostician but didn't know how to be polite. We decided to go to this doctor anyway. He *was* excellent, but it was also true that he had no bedside manner. We decided that was acceptable, since we weren't looking for a friend, just a good doctor. If you find yourself in this kind of situation, decide what is important to you. You are the only one who knows what you need and want from your doctor.

Another form of rude behavior in doctors is keeping you waiting when you have an appointment, but sometimes this situation must be tolerated. You have to remember, if *you* think your doctor is great, others probably feel the same way, so be prepared to wait. If you need to be out by a certain time, call the doctor's office in advance to see if this will be possible. Remind the receptionist when you arrive that you must be out by a certain time. If you can, book the first appointment of the day, the first appointment after lunch, or the last appointment of the day. Call the doctor's office before you leave for your appointment and see if the doctor's schedule is running on time.

My oncologist always ran one to two hours late. His nurses and patients were aware of this. Most of the time, nothing could be done about the situation because there were always emergencies that had to be handled. But I found that the nurses were upset with the patients because they never complained to the doctor about being kept waiting. Instead, they tended to blame the nurses for what was happening. And so the nurses worked under more and more stress.

If your doctor keeps you waiting consistently and you don't want to change doctors, tell him that this is a concern of yours and ask how it could be remedied.

Your Doctor Has a Bad Attitude

With more people viewing the doctor-patient relationship as a consumer issue, patients are beginning to realize that they don't have to put up with a doctor who has a bad attitude. If you have a doctor who seems mean and surly, *find a new doctor.* You have many to choose from.

Your Doctor Doesn't Take Enough Time with You

Do you always feel rushed when you're at the doctor's? Do you feel that you never get a chance to say what you wanted to, your questions don't get answered, or you don't even get a chance to ask them? Perhaps your doctor's staff is overscheduling his day. Managed-care and HMO doctors make more money by treating more patients. This usually doesn't cause too much of a problem except when everyone gets sick at the same time. So it's up to you to make sure you are getting the time you need.

When making your appointment, tell the nurse or receptionist that you want some extra time with the doctor. Scheduling nurses often complain that patients do not say what they are coming in for. The patient may say on the phone that she thinks she has the flu, but once she is with the doctor, she starts discussing the severe chest pains she's had for the past six months. You have every right to discuss your condition fully with your doctor, but try to let the nurse know your concerns so she will be able to schedule the doctor's time more effectively.

Your Doctor Is Unwilling to Discuss the Diagnosis Fully

There is no reason why a doctor shouldn't discuss her diagnosis with you, but she may be reticent. Perhaps she's not sure you can handle the truth. This kind of problem may be more common among older doctors who weren't trained in the current era of openness. If you feel that information is being withheld from you, tell the doctor that you want to know everything. It is not up to the doctor to withhold information from you. If you *don't* want to be told the complete diagnosis, have the doctor discuss it openly with a family member or close friend. Remember, if your doctor doesn't change, *change doctors.*

Your Doctor Ignores Your Concerns

The most important thing to remember regarding your health care is that you know your body better than anyone. You know when you're not feeling right.

A thirty-year-old woman I interviewed went to her doctor asking for a mammogram. She explained her family's long history of breast cancer and said she was concerned that she might be susceptible. Due to insurance restrictions, her doctor refused her requests, stating that the literature showed there was no advantage to having a mammogram so early. The doctor told her not to worry; nothing was wrong.

This woman was smart enough to seek out another doctor who wouldn't ignore her. She had her mammogram, and a small lump was discovered.

Rely on your own instincts about how you're feeling. If your doctor ignores your concerns, *change doctors.*

You Lose Trust in Your Doctor

Never stay with a doctor you don't trust. A thirty-year-old woman who attended one of my lectures told of the problems she and her husband had encountered while trying to get pregnant. They had been trying for six months, with no results. Her obstetrician informed her that unless she had three different procedures done within the next three months, the last one major surgery, she would never have a baby. The doctor's attitude, along with his refusal to discuss alternative treatments, caused her to lose trust in his diagnosis. There are many excellent doctors practicing medicine, and there is no reason to stay with someone you don't trust.

Your Doctor Objects to You Seeking a Second Opinion

Most insurance plans *require* you to seek a second opinion when you are considering surgery or other extensive treatment. Since this is an established practice, most doctors have no problem with it. But sometimes a doctor may consider a patient seeking a second opinion to be questioning his knowledge and ability.

When you are looking for a doctor to consult for that second opinion, don't ask your current doctor for a referral. You may get a friend of the doctor's who is eager to confirm his buddy's diagnosis. Call the charge nurse on the surgery floor of your local hospital, or ask the nurses in your current doctor's office for some names. In short, choose the second-opinion doctor as thoroughly as you chose the first.

Twice when I went to get second opinions, I ended up staying with the doctor who had given me the second opinion. Don't look at the second opinion as a necessary evil. You may find yourself with a reason to *change doctors.*

Your Doctor Leaves Her Current Practice

If your doctor leaves her current practice and you choose not to go with her or are not able to, it's time to *change doctors.* There are many reasons a doctor may leave her practice: for example, she may move out of the area, or maybe she leaves medicine for a new field. Whatever the reason, you still need to *find a new doctor.* If you like this doctor and are happy with the care you have received, ask her to recommend a new doctor.

Your Doctor Retires

When my oncologist retired, I was once again in the position of looking for a new doctor. Unlike similar situations I had been in, this was more difficult. I was finishing my treatment for cancer and had a strong emotional attachment to this doctor. He had followed me through my whole experience, and I wasn't thrilled with the thought of starting all over again with someone who was going to relate to me as little more than a new patient. But I had no choice. I asked my oncologist whom he recommended as a good doctor for me. I then met with the new doctor. I am now satisfied with this new doctor-patient relationship.

When replacing a retiring doctor, look for one who won't be retiring or leaving her practice any time soon. An important aspect of your health care should be a close, ongoing relationship with your doctors.

Make sure that your medical records are forwarded whenever you start seeing a new doctor or a specialist or when you move to a new town. It is important that your new doctor know about your past medical history. This knowledge is essential in putting together a complete treatment plan.

Chapter 5

The Health-Care Consumer and Other Health-Care Providers

Health care encompasses far more than just the doctor-patient relationship. Throughout the course of your life you will have to have tests and procedures done. Some, like blood tests, hearing tests, pregnancy tests, and blood pressure monitoring, will be carried out in your doctor's office. Others, such as mammograms, X rays, or MRIs, may be done in labs. You may even require a biopsy or monitoring that includes a stay in the hospital, where you will have countless encounters with technicians, nurses, and pharmacists. Your relationship with these health-care professionals is just as important as your relationship with your doctor.

Hospitals

It may seem that you are required to give up your freedom of choice, along with your dignity, the moment you check in at the hospital admission office, but it doesn't have to be that way. You and your doctor work as a team in the doctor's office, and it is even more important that you carry this team relationship over to your stay in the hospital.

Choosing a Hospital

The choice of which hospital you enter is not entirely up to you. Your doctor must have privileges at a hospital to be able to admit you there. "Having privileges" means the doctor is on the hospital's staff. This is a reciprocal agreement: The hospital allows the doctor to practice there and the doctor helps fill up the hospital's beds. Most doctors have privileges at more than one hospital, so together you and your doctor can decide where you will receive the best care. In addition to choosing a hospital where your doctor can practice, you will want to choose the one that will best be able to handle your condition. You may also want to consider a hospital that is close to your home, so it will be more convenient for your family to visit you.

There are different kinds of hospitals: "specialty" hospitals such as pediatric or orthopedic, and medical-surgical hospitals. Although you might want to choose a hospital that specializes in your particular ailment, you will get more complete care in a medical-surgical hospital should complications arise that are not connected to your original diagnosis.

You will also want to consider medical centers that are associated with a university. Teaching hospitals, community hospitals, nonprofit hospitals, and for-profit hospitals are all options. Most insurance plans have a specific list of hospitals their subscribers can use.

University medical centers are usually in the forefront of medical research. If you have an unusual illness or are going to have experimental surgery or treatment, this may be the kind of hospital for you. Top-notch doctors and surgeons flock to these hospitals to have the chance to do ground-breaking research. The problem is, you will rarely get the chance to see these doctors or have them work on you. In university medical centers, educating medical students is as important as caring for patients. The patients are there for the students' convenience. You will not find continuity of care; there is a constant flow of doctors in and out.

The cost of a stay in a teaching hospital will be high, sometimes twice as much as in other hospitals. Medical students' salaries need to be paid and the newest equipment needs to be bought and maintained. Also, there are many nonpaying patients whose conditions make great test cases for the students' education.

If your doctor and you come to the conclusion that a teaching hospital is where you will receive the best medical treatment, realize that this will not be a restful and relaxing experience, nor will you be getting the personalized care you could expect in a smaller hospital. In teaching hospitals more tests and procedures are done, for the students want to make sure they come up with the right diagnosis. They also make sure they have a paper record of the medical care provided to protect against possible lawsuits.

For-profit hospitals tend to be costly as well. In addition to paying hospital staff, for-profit hospitals have to make sure their stockholders get a good return on their money. You won't necessarily experience a higher standard of care in a for-profit hospital, but you may have plusher surroundings. Advertisements for these hospitals tend to emphasize private rooms, gourmet meals, and birth and labor suites. The thought is that these special touches will make a hospital stay more tolerable.

It was originally predicted that for-profit hospitals would help bring down the cost of health care. In most businesses, competition means lower cost to the public.

This has not proven true with hospitals, however. The medical community has just continued with business as usual.

You will want to question the hospitals you are considering. Make sure that there is a doctor in-house, in addition to the emergency room doctor, twenty-four hours a day. This arrangement is not required in many states. But a hospital without a doctor on call full time is little more than a very expensive hotel.

The Caregiving Team

Once you are in the hospital, you will be relying on far more people than your personal physician to take care of you. Here are descriptions of some of the other health-care professionals who staff hospitals.

Doctors

Included in this catch-all category are residents, interns, and medical students. In a teaching hospital, you will most likely have contact with all of them on a daily basis. During "rounds," the patients become the subject matter of the day. Generally, doctors in training tend to ignore the patient and conduct the discussion as though they were dealing not with a real live human being but just a medical condition. Here is your chance to further the cause of doctor-patient relations in the future. Don't let the doctors treat you like an object. When they ask you questions, make sure you have eye contact before you answer them. When they refer to you as "the knee in room 503," introduce yourself to them and ask them to do the same. The future patients of these doctors will appreciate your lesson in patient relations.

In most teaching hospitals, all "doctors," whether they are residents or medical students, are referred to as "Doctor." When someone comes into your room, ask what his position is. If he is a medical student and you don't feel comfortable with him handling your case, tell him this and request a resident. This holds true *whenever* you don't feel comfortable with someone handling your case. Maybe you have a specialist who treats you with no respect or acts as if you aren't there at all. Discuss this problem with your doctor. There could be a particular reason he wants the specialist on the case. If not, get someone else.

A man in one of my seminars had the misfortune of dealing with an impaired doctor. In this case the doctor had been drinking heavily, and his condition was a secret to no one. It was late at night, and it looked as though this gentleman would have to have emergency surgery. The impaired doctor was on call for surgery. Luckily, it turned out that the surgery was not required, but this man said he didn't know what he would have done if it had been necessary! If this should happen to you, *refuse* to have the doctor operate. Don't become the willing victim of a tragic mistake. Insist that a *qualified* doctor be found *immediately*. If you have to, start screaming *lawsuit* and you'll find people moving awfully fast to make things right.

If you are scheduling an elective surgery and plan to be admitted to a teaching hospital, don't do it in July. July is when the new interns and medical students start.

If you are scheduling an elective surgery and plan to be admitted to a teaching hospital, don't do it in July. July is when the new interns and medical students start. They are ready and eager to meet and cure their first willing patient.

Nurses

Nurses are in charge of your day-to-day care in the hospital. The title *nurse* in the hospital, like *doctor,* covers many different categories: registered nurse (R.N.), licensed practical nurse (L.P.N.), nurse's aide, nursing student, and orderly. You will have primary nurses who are responsible for your overall care. The relationship between these nurses and you is very important. If for some reason you don't get along, ask for different primary nurses. I have found that if you make the nurse your friend, she or he will have a vested interest in your well-being.

Although the nurses will be in charge of your care, it is important for you to know what is being done and to still ask questions. If you have drug allergies, make sure that the nurse is aware of them and that they are listed on the front of your chart. I am allergic to iodine and, since it is an antiseptic widely used in hospitals, the nurse wrote this information on signs and posted them on the door to my room and on the wall over my bed. This way, if technicians came in to take blood while I was asleep, they would see the signs and make sure iodine was not used.

Know what you're taking. When the nurse brings medications in for you, ask what they are, why they were prescribed, and what side effects, if any, you should be aware of. Since the staff on your hospital floor changes frequently, it is important that you understand what is being prescribed and what your doctor has recommended for your treatment. This way, you can be a backup to the nurses and lessen the chance of mistakes being made in your hospital care. If your nurse is defensive and uncomfortable with your taking an active role in your care, ask for a change of nurses.

I have learned a lot from nurses in the hospital. When I had major surgery and was about to be released, my primary nurse asked me if I had been given a shot to prevent pneumonia. I had never even heard of this shot, but it turned out that it was an extremely important treatment for me to receive. I was very thankful that my nurse asked about this.

There were many other situations in which nurses were a great help in my recovery. When I woke up from major surgery, my nurse gave me his watch so that I would know when it was time to self-administer my pain medication. I've had nurses come into my room at three o'clock in the morning when I was feeling lonely, just to sit and keep me company. I've had a nurse come in after a roomful of obnoxious medical students had left and tell me I had the right to ask them to leave my room and to leave me alone. I have been very lucky in some of the nurses I've had.

On the other hand, I had a nurse who, when I was in terrible pain, told me that I would get pain medication when she was "good and ready and not before."

When I was having a drug reaction in the hospital and wanted to see a doctor, my nurse told me I was crazy. She refused to waste a doctor's time by having him come to see me. She told me to stop acting like a "baby" and to "shut up." Luckily my sister called during this discussion; when I yelled into the phone that they were going to let me die there, a doctor was called in. It turned out I was having a severe reaction to a painkiller. The doctor asked the nurse several times why he hadn't been called earlier. Don't hold the mistaken belief that, just because you're in the hospital and these are health-care professionals, they know what is best for you.

Many hospitals are finding it cost-effective to employ more nurses' aides and fewer nurses. Although this practice will save money because nurses' aides earn about half as much as nurses, the quality of care you receive may be compromised. If you are not happy with the care you are receiving, complain! It is the responsibility of the hospital to ensure that quality care is provided.

Laboratory Technicians

Lab technicians are necessary evils in the hospital. They will come in the middle of the night to take your blood. They will come with a wheelchair at the crack of dawn to take you for X rays. Lab technicians in the hospital are not accustomed to dealing with patients on a personal level. Rarely will they introduce themselves and tell you why they are there and what needs to be done.

I had a technician who saw nothing wrong with poking me three or four times to find a vein so that he could take blood. When that technician came back the next day, I told him to send in someone else who would do it right the first time. He was shocked. Then he told me that I had no other choice. I called my nurse into the room, and she was able to find someone else.

When I was admitted to the hospital in an emergency while undergoing chemotherapy, I was subjected to outright rudeness by a lab technician. Like a lot of oncology patients, I had lost most of my hair. When the technician came in to do a test, she looked at me and said, "Boy, is that short hair! I would never wear *my* hair like *that!*"

One day when I was undergoing radiation therapy, the lab technician seemed to have great fun inviting students, aides, and interns into the room to see what was going on. After my treatment was over, I told her never to have anyone else come into the room like that again unless I was asked permission.

If you are uncomfortable with a lab technician of the opposite sex, ask for one of the same sex. This is your right as a health-care consumer.

These examples merely underline the fact that doctors aren't gods, nurses aren't angels, and lab technicians are unavoidable. Sometimes they make mistakes. But that doesn't mean that you have to put up with them. There is a way of dealing with these problems.

Patient Representatives

Every hospital employs someone whose job includes mediating patients' concerns. This is the person you should contact when you have problems with hospital personnel. The ideal solution would be to deal with the problematic person directly. But if that doesn't work, or you don't want to talk with the offender, contact the hospital's patient representative. It is the representative's job to see that problems the patient encounters in the hospital are handled quickly and effectively.

You Are in Control

What the previous examples add up to is the recognition that, even though you are sick and in the hospital, you don't have to give up your right to be a partner in your care. What you want to do instead is let other people deal with the unimportant things. *Your* job is to concentrate on getting better. That's not always easy in a hospital. Hospital surroundings, schedules, rules, and regulations are all put together for the benefit of the people who work there, not for the people who are treated there. But this doesn't mean that you have to conform to all their requirements. You're the one who's paying. Do what will work best for *you*.

Start looking out for your needs before you are even admitted to the hospital. Call the admission office about a week before your stay is planned and ask if you can fill out the admission papers over the phone or pick them up to fill them out in advance. This way you will not have to sit and wait on the day you are admitted. If a staff member tells you, "We just don't do that," let him know you'd like him to try. This procedure is commonly used with obstetric patients planning to have their babies in the hospital. Screaming women in labor sitting in the hospital lobby wouldn't instill much faith in that facility.

Read the consent forms before you sign them. The forms are all worded to protect the hospital and its staff from any problems that may occur. One of the forms I was asked to sign stated that should one of the health-care workers get stuck by a needle while performing a procedure on me, he or she would have access to all my medical records. I changed this statement to add that I would have access to the health-care worker's medical records as well. There may be things that you don't want to consent to. Talk to your doctor about having them omitted. Make sure you initial any changes you make to the forms.

Many hospitals will ask for payment in advance. If you have health insurance there is no reason for this requirement. I refuse to pay in advance. I figure they have to make *sure* they take good care of me in the hospital in order to get paid. My husband tells me that I'm superstitious, but it's always worked for me!

Once you're in the hospital, there are several things you can do to make your stay more pleasant. First, don't bring a lot of things from home. Many people will be coming in and out of your room, and you won't be in your room all the time, so there is not much security. Do bring some pictures from home. I always brought a photograph of my husband and newborn daughter with me, as well as one of me with my parents, sister, and brother. In addition to cheering me up when I was feeling down, the photographs enabled the hospital staff to see me as a real person and not just a disease.

Ask if you can wear your own nightclothes. If this is not possible, wear two hospital gowns: one backward and then one forward over it, like a robe. Although dignity in a hospital is a rarity, it's not impossible.

Make sure that the telephone works, as well as the nurses' call button. Many patients will tell you that their call button didn't work because the nurses never responded to it. It could be, however, that the nurses heard the call but decided they would respond when they wanted to. If you have a difficult time getting a nurse to come to your room and you need one in an emergency, call the hospital operator on the phone, tell her your room number, and say you need help.

You can *always* get a nurse to come to your room if you push the nurses' call button in the bathroom. The nurse will have to come into your room to turn off the alarm; it can't be turned off from the nurses' station.

Most of all, make the best of a not-so-good situation. Face it—the hospital is not a hotel. No matter how much you are paying for your accommodations, you'll never confuse the memory of your stay with even the worst of resort vacations. But you *can* improve *some* of the conditions while you are there. If you have a window in your room, open the curtains and let the daylight in. If fluorescent lights give you a headache, turn them off and have the nurse bring in a lamp. If you have a roommate who is noisy, who has parties, or who is constantly on the phone, ask to be moved to another room because he is interfering with your recovery. If blood is being taken from you four to five times a day, talk to the nurse about having it done less frequently. If you are being given drugs you

> *You can always get a nurse to come to your room if you push the nurses' call button in the bathroom. The nurse will have to come into your room to turn off the alarm; it can't be turned off from the nurses' station.*

don't want, like sleeping pills, refuse them and make sure you will not be charged for what you don't take.

And, whatever you do, don't accept treatments just because "That's the way we do things."

To get the quality care you require in the hospital, you need the hospital staff on your side. When my dad had surgery, I brought the nurses on his floor gourmet cookies. Some people say you shouldn't have to do that. You're paying for your care—*demand* what you want! But basically I'm a realist. If I'm scheduled for surgery, I'm not about to demand anything from someone who will be cutting into me. I would rather have him laugh at my jokes, enjoy my cookies, and realize what a terrific person I am.

Special Needs

If you have special needs, make sure they will be met. If your hearing or sight is impaired, discuss this problem with your nurse. How should she get your attention when she comes into the room? Should she touch you or gently shake the bed rail? Write this information down and post it on your door so hospital personnel will know. Want to make sure your family can visit? Post pictures of them on your door so that they will have no problem going into your room. If you don't want visitors, let that be known as well.

Since you are not always at your best in the hospital, it may be a great help to have a family member or friend with you. If you are not able to speak up for yourself, that person will. Make sure that the staff realizes that your helper is speaking on your behalf. This is extremely important for parents with kids in the hospital. Discuss staying with your child in the hospital with the doctor beforehand; then let the nurses know that you will be there whenever your child asks you to be.

Many times in the hospital I've been told, "We'll have to call your doctor if you want to do that." When I've said, "Fine. In fact, I'll call him right now," suddenly the nurses didn't want to interrupt him and found a way to do what I had asked. Don't let hospital personnel intimidate you.

Pharmacists

Not many people would think to include the pharmacist as a member of the health-care team. The doctor is the one who prescribes the medications and their dosages and gives directions for their use. The pharmacist, you may think, is merely the person who hands over the pills after you've waited in line at the drugstore for way too long.

But health-care consumers know that the relationship with the pharmacist can be just as important as the relationship with the doctor. A Gallup poll discovered that Americans believe pharmacists are the most honest and ethical professionals, ahead of lawyers, the clergy, and doctors.[1] Whereas your doctor will prescribe medications for specific illnesses or injuries as they occur, if you regularly patronize one drugstore the pharmacist will have a complete record of your drug-taking history, including which drugs you are allergic to. He also has access to information about possible interactions between drugs you are taking together at any given time. Take advantage of your pharmacist's knowledge. In medical school, your doctor took one semester's worth of drug-related courses

---

[1]Leslie McAneny, "Pharmacists Retain Wide Lead as Most Honorable Profession," *The Gallup Poll Monthly,* July 1993, p. 37.

to learn about prescribing types and dosages of drugs. Pharmacists spend three years learning what they need to know on the same subject.

A recent survey by the Coalition for Consumer Access to Pharmaceutical Care showed that 88 percent of Americans see pharmacists as their primary or secondary source of information on drugs, although 43 percent had not talked with the pharmacist about their last prescription.[2]

In fact, eleven percent of hospital admissions are due to patients taking their drugs improperly.

It's striking that up to 50 percent of prescriptions dispensed each year are taken incorrectly. In fact, eleven percent of hospital admissions are due to patients taking their drugs improperly. If you are unsure about the directions given by your doctor for your new prescription, ask the pharmacist for help.

Drug Interactions and Side Effects

Ask questions of your pharmacist when you are given a new prescription. How will this medication interact with the other drugs you are taking? Make sure you mention all the over-the-counter drugs you are taking, including vitamins and minerals. If you have drug allergies or sensitivities, ask if this prescription is something to be concerned about. The pharmacist will also be able to tell you about interactions between drugs and foods.

Drug Interactions
- If you are taking antibiotics and a contraceptive pill together, the Pill won't work.

[2]Coalition for Consumer Access to Pharmaceutical Care. Press release June 1, 1994.

- Epilepsy drugs interfere with the Pill.
- If you take the heart medication Lanoxin and then eat oatmeal, the drug won't work.
- Drinking grapefruit juice can cause high levels of certain drugs (Seldane, Procardia, Plendil) to build up in your bloodstream, with drastic results.
- You can become addicted to nasal spray and OTC eyedrops that clear up redness. Using them regularly causes a rebound effect—i.e., a worsening of the symptoms. You'll have to use more, and more and the symptoms will keep returning.
- Taking decongestants raises your blood pressure.
- Over-the-counter allergy, cold, and cough medicines may exaggerate the effects of Valium.
- Taking estrogen will affect your thyroid level in blood tests.
- Tetracycline should not be taken with dairy products; they diminish its effectiveness.
- You should not drink alcohol if you are taking tranquilizers, sedatives, antidepressants, or painkillers.
- Smoking and taking oral contraceptives increases the risk of heart attack and stroke.
- Smoking while wearing a nicotine patch can cause heart palpitations and even death.
- Antacids, most of which contain high levels of sodium, could be dangerous for those with high blood pressure or heart trouble or for those on low-salt diets.
- You should not mix antacids containing aluminum with orange juice, for this mixture increases the absorption of aluminum in the body by as much as ten times. Wait two to three hours

after taking antacids before eating or drinking citrus products.

- You should not take Vitamin C and aspirin together. Heavy doses could cause ulcers.

Whenever a new drug is prescribed for you, let the pharmacist know of any unusual eating habits you have, in addition to all the other drugs you are taking. Do you eat a pound of broccoli every day? Do you eat natural black licorice? Don't keep it a secret. It may affect how your medications will work.

In addition to drug-food interactions, you also need to watch out for drug side effects. Some may be so mild that you'll attribute them to something else, but be aware of what's happening to your body when you are taking medications.

Dry eyes, dry mouth, sleeplessness, irritability, dizziness, blurred vision, and nausea are all side effects of different drugs. If you have any of these symptoms while taking drugs, let your doctor know. Some side effects you will be able to put up with. Others can be alleviated by changing the dosage or type of medication.

Side Effects
- Some sleeping pills stay in your bloodstream for a long time. Be aware of slowed reflexes and drowsiness, especially when driving.
- It is possible to overdose on vitamins. There is no reason to take more than the recommended daily allowance unless your doctor specifically prescribes it.
- Even if you've taken a medication for years, you could still have a reaction to it.

- Reactions don't always happen right away! A reaction may come on slowly, taking weeks or months.
- Less than 5 percent of drug reactions get reported to the drug companies and the Food and Drug Administration (FDA). Make sure you tell your doctor and that he informs the drug company and the proper health agencies about any drug reactions you have.

Patients will sometimes see new drug side effects as additional symptoms of the original ailment. They may end up taking many medications at the same time to combat all the side effects. The health-care consumer knows that the job of medication is to cure illness. This purpose is defeated when drugs are taken to cure the side effects of other drugs.

Chapter 6

Saving Money

Health care is expensive. This is not news to anyone. If you read the newspaper or watch television, you know how much medical care costs the American public. Employers, insurance companies, and doctors, as well as the general public, are all interested in spending less to stay healthy. Employers want to know when their premiums will go down. Managed-care organizations state that price is the most important consideration in the health care they deliver. Doctors and nurses are spending more of their time arguing with insurance officials over what medical procedures should be covered and how long patients can remain in the hospital. The quality of care that patients receive is at stake.

Many people feel that Americans will have to learn to live with a lower level of health care. It is the job of the health-care consumer to get the best-quality care and still save money. This won't always be easy. You will have to insist that your health-care providers not think of cost before care. This doesn't mean that quality care must cost more, just that the quality of the care provided must be considered first. Then ways must be found to provide that care in an economical manner.

Some costly treatments may end up saving money in the long run. The health-care consumer–doctor team does not just look at short-term remedies, it is aware of long-term consequences. Some people suggest that you are being less than a good consumer if you are not constantly questioning your doctor about the cost and necessity of diagnostic tests, X rays, treatments, and procedures. I am not a doctor. I have worked hard and have put a great deal of research into finding and choosing my doctors. I rely on my doctors' education and experience to dictate what should be done, though I still question them when I feel too many tests or procedures are being performed.

Prevention

Our health-care system seems to encourage us to delay getting medical care. Most insurance plans will not pay for annual physicals, routine immunizations, or regular check-ups. Therefore most people don't go to the doctor until they're really sick. But more and more health insurance companies are beginning to see how expensive it can be to get a sick person well and how much cheaper it can be to keep people well in the first place. Managed-care organizations have found that it is far more cost-effective to pay for a flu shot than to intervene after the flu has become pneumonia.

Wellness, Not Illness

Not only has wellness become a prudent health-care goal, it's also big business. Wellness programs are currently being promoted by employers and hospitals as well as by insurance companies. These companies are concerned about their employees' well-being, but they're also seeing benefits to their bottom line. Employees become healthier, they miss less work, and the time they put in at work produces better results.

Hospitals are offering wellness classes for their employees and for the community at large, and they are seeing direct improvements in their bottom line. The money they make from their wellness programs makes up for some of the money they've lost to shorter and shorter hospital stays. The best proof that these programs are making an impact is the fact that insurance companies have been lowering their premiums for companies that have initiated wellness programs.

The idea behind wellness programs is preventive care. Physical fitness is encouraged for all ages, and programs for addiction treatments, smoking cessation, and weight loss are available at hospitals and in community programs. In some companies and hospitals there are stress-management seminars, back care classes, aerobics classes, and basketball courts. You can also find some alternative choices like belly dancing, meditation classes, and yoga. Most wellness programs also include free tests for cholesterol and high blood pressure.

I think it's wonderful that people are concentrating on being and staying healthy. Do be aware, though, that many of these services are not provided solely from altruistic motives. Hospitals provide exercise classes to keep you well, but they are hoping that you will avail yourself of their services if you *do* get sick. When you go to get free health-screening tests, should your results not be in the normal range, you will be referred to doctors practicing at the hospital that sponsors these free tests. That is fine if there is truly something wrong, but the quality of these test results can sometimes be questionable. Ask the people running the tests how many false positives they encounter. Remember, these programs are not always being done just for the public good. In some cases their purpose is to drum up future business.

Stress Reduction

Another way of preventing illness is to reduce the stress in your life. Stress can cause many problems, including illness. Managing stress can play a tremendous role in preventing heart attacks. Although "reduce your stress" is a popular catch phrase with doctors these days and seems almost impossible to do successfully, there are concrete ways of dealing with stress that you can fit into your everyday life.

- Exercise regularly
- Spend time with your friends
- Get a pet
- Keep your immunizations current—tetanus, flu, pneumonia
- Take a vacation—hotels are a lot cheaper and more fun than hospitals
- Get enough sleep
- Learn to say no
- Take a hot bath
- Get a massage
- Have a sense of humor about things

Even if you don't incorporate all of these options into your life, putting a couple of them into action can reduce your stress.

Getting the Most
for Your Prescription Dollar

The money spent on prescription drugs is a big part of the American health-care dollar. Some people have found their own way of saving money when it comes to pre-scriptions. Their erroneous money-saving tips include not filling the doctor's prescription, filling the prescription but taking only half the medicine called for and saving the other half for the next time it's needed, or taking a friend's or family member's prescription instead. Unfortunately, all of these "solutions" defeat the health-care consumer's goal of getting quality care while saving money. None of these practices will get you well. In fact, they can make you sicker. Some better choices for saving money are described in the following sections.

Use Generic Drugs

Almost 40 percent of prescriptions today are filled with generic drugs. You may have little or no choice in this matter, since most insurance companies will not cover the cost of name-brand drugs unless the doctor specifically prescribes them. When your doctor prescribes medicine for you, be sure to ask if the generic is all right for you to take. Both doctors and consumers seem a bit wary when it comes to using generic drugs—and with good reason. In 1989, some may remember, generic drug companies submitted falsified data and some FDA offi-cials took bribes from generic companies whose drugs were being reviewed. The review process is said to have been improved, but there are still problems found in generic drugs.

The *Wall Street Journal* reported that in early 1994, problems were found in some asthma drugs. Patients who took the name-brand drug Proventil found that their con-dition improved. Those who were switched to the generic equivalent, Albuterol, got worse. The generic was recalled in January 1994 when bacterial contamination was found in it.[1] It's alleged that about one hundred people died from using Albuterol.

Overall, generic drugs are a cost-effective choice. If you have a sensitivity to many drugs, ask your doctor to prescribe the name brand. When I was in chemotherapy I wanted to make sure that I was receiving the correct drugs. Since these were all drugs I hadn't taken before, I had my doctor prescribe the name brand. If your doctor states that he would prefer you take the name brand, ask him to prescribe that brand by name.

Did you know that different generic versions of the same drug may differ in quality? A young woman in one of my seminars had taken a painkiller for some time and it had worked well. One time, however, after she had had the prescription refilled, she found that her pain was not being relieved. She called her pharmacist and told him. He said the company that had been manufacturing the generic drug she had been taking had stopped production and that the new generic, from another company, wasn't as effective. He suggested that, although it would cost her more money, she should get her prescription filled with the name-brand drug. She called her doctor, explained the situation, and asked him to write her a new prescription for the name-brand drug. Now she has medicine that works and her insurance still covers the cost.

Beware when the pharmacist asks you if you want to switch to another drug that is *almost* the same as what your doctor has prescribed. He may tell you that it's a lot cheaper than the original drug prescribed. What he may not tell you is that he makes more money from the drug he is suggesting. Stick with your doctor's choice!

---

[1]*Wall Street Journal,* February 2, 1995, pp. A1, A12.

Start Prescriptions with a Small Amount of Pills

With so many drugs to choose from, it's not always easy for the doctor to prescribe the right drug to help you. If you're like me, you may be sensitive to several drugs. Ask your doctor, when he is giving you a new drug, to prescribe a small number of pills with a full refill option. Although this will probably cost you more per pill, if it turns out you won't be taking the full prescription, you won't have spent money on pills you have to throw out.

Buy More Pills at One Time

If you are taking the same medicine on an ongoing basis, you may be able to get a better price if you buy a couple of months' worth of pills at one time. Ask your pharmacist if there is a price break when you buy more pills—making sure that you will be able to use the pills you buy before their expiration date. There is no savings if you can't use up the medicine before it expires.

Mail-Order Companies

Some insurance companies are trying to promote drugs-by-mail programs. If you have a standard monthly prescription to fill, you may be able to achieve great savings this way, while still using your local pharmacy for prescriptions that need to be filled immediately.

For those who wear contact lenses, buying through mail order is also a way to save money. You may run into an obstacle here, though. In order to buy contact lenses through the mail, you need to send in a doctor's prescription. Doctors frequently refuse to give patients copies of contact lens prescriptions. They will tell you that this is

Ask your doctor, when he is giving you a new drug, to prescribe a small number of pills with a full refill option. Although this will probably cost you more per pill, if it turns out you won't be taking the full prescription, you won't have spent money on pills you have to throw out.

because the lenses need to be professionally fitted and checked to see that the prescription has been filled correctly. This may be part of the reason; the other part is that there is very little money in eye exams, and far more in the selling of contact lenses.

Make Sure You Get the Amount of Medicine You Pay For

In one of my seminars a gentleman said he'd just refilled a prescription for a painkiller. When he got home from the pharmacy, his doctor called him and told him he was using the medicine too often and should make an appointment to come in. The man, knowing he was taking the medicine as directed, decided to count the pills in the prescription he had just picked up. The prescription was for thirty pills, but the man counted only twenty-three. When he called the pharmacy to complain they didn't even question the amount the man had found. They told him to come in any time to get the seven missing pills.

Although this may sound like nit-picking, when some pills sell for over a dollar each, a big loss can add up over the long term.

Ask Your Doctor for Samples

Whenever your doctor prescribes a medicine for you, ask if he has any samples. My current internist gives out samples regularly. When I take my daughter to the doctor and something is prescribed for her, I ask about samples. Most of the time, I find the doctor will give me one or two. In addition to being able to start the prescription immediately, getting samples solves the problem of having to wait at the pharmacy with a screaming child in tow until the prescription is ready. (When you must pick up a prescription, have the doctor's office call it in to the pharmacy for you. The medicine will be ready when you get there.)

When getting samples from your doctor, make sure you receive the same information you would have gotten had you bought the prescription at your pharmacy. Find out when to take the medicine, how often to take it, how to take it (with food, without food, with water, etc.), and how long to take it. Ask if you should be aware of any potential side effects, and make sure that your doctor knows of all the other medicines you are taking at the same time. Doctors' samples, when taken properly, can be a great money saver!

Don't Insist That Your Doctor Prescribe Drugs

Everyone is looking for the wonder pill that will make them feel better instantly. Not wanting to miss work, getting ready to go on vacation, or having to take care of sick kids are great reasons not to be laid up in bed for several days with a cold. Unfortunately, sometimes a cold is just a cold. It is not an infection that antibiotics will cure or a flu that you could have prevented with a flu shot.

Many doctors find themselves faced with patients who relentlessly insist that they prescribe antibiotics for what they know is just a cold. Don't demand that your doctor prescribe drugs that won't work. In the long run this practice causes more problems than it solves. And you will be spending money needlessly.

Use Prescription Instead of Over-the-Counter Drugs

More and more former prescription drugs are now available over the counter. In addition to not being covered by health insurance, these OTC drugs may not be the same strength as the prescription drug was. Ask your doctor to prescribe a drug instead. You'll get the proper dosage, insurance will cover it, and you will be better able to keep unwanted drug interactions under control.

Consumers are not the only ones who benefit from the different ways to save on prescription drugs. Some drug manufacturers offer pharmacists rewards for pushing their brand: cash for every prescription that gets switched to a different brand. All the pharmacist has to do is show proof that your prescription was changed from a competitor's brand. The bonus, per prescription, can reach as high as $35.[2] The drug companies see this as simply reimbursing pharmacists for doing their part in reducing overall prescription drug costs.

Some see this practice as legally questionable. I think the chance of reducing prescription drug costs would be better if the bonuses were given to the consumer paying for the drug and not the pharmacist dispensing it.

Getting Your Money's Worth

Sometimes the treatments prescribed by your doctor will be expensive. Make sure you get what you are paying for. Recently a scheme by a contact lens company came to light. This manufacturer markets contact lenses that can be used for a week or two and then thrown away; lenses that can be used up to three months; and lenses that last up to a year. These various lenses cost anywhere from around

---

[2]David France, "The New Drug Money," *Redbook*, January 1995, p. 86.

eight dollars a pair up to several hundred dollars a pair. The problem is that the exact same lenses were being packaged and sold in different ways. Talk to your doctor; ask *him* about the differences between medical products and how best to spend your money.

Ways to Save in Hospitals

Hospital care is *very* expensive. Although there may be alternatives to a hospital stay, there are times when your doctor will insist that you be admitted to the hospital for the care you require. So let's look at a few ways to save money when you're facing a stay in the hospital.

Preadmission Tests

Hospitals require that preadmission tests be performed on patients coming into the hospital for surgery and other medical procedures. These tests may include chest X rays, blood tests, and an EKG. Ask your doctor about having these tests performed *before* you enter the hospital, at an outside laboratory. The cost of tests done at the hospital, instead of at an independent lab, can be as much as eight times higher. Most hospitals require that these tests be done two to three days before surgery; discuss scheduling restrictions with your doctor.

Required Medications

We have all heard horror stories of hospitals charging three dollars for a single aspirin. Some people might think, "What's the big deal? Hospitals have to make money somehow." But if you're paying three dollars for that aspirin, that's the same as going to your local drugstore and paying

Ask your doctor about having these tests performed before you enter the hospital, at an outside laboratory. The cost of tests done at the hospital, instead of at an independent lab, can be as much as eight times higher.

three hundred dollars for a 100-tablet bottle of Excedrin. That sort of puts things in perspective, doesn't it?

Talk to your doctor and see if it would be possible to bring in some of your own things. If you take certain prescription drugs on an ongoing basis, ask if you can bring them with you. There are good reasons for hospitals not wanting patients to bring in their own medicines; they have no quality control. You may have a reaction to something you're taking and the nursing staff won't be sure if it was something they gave you or something you took on your own. Ask your doctor about bringing your own prescriptions in and having the nurses dispense them. This way they will know exactly what it is you're taking and when you're taking it.

When you start talking to your doctor and the hospital staff about doing some of these things you will probably be told, "That's not the way we do things here." Don't be afraid to let them know that you would like to try a new way. If your doctor supports you in your decision, there is no reason why the hospital can't go along as well.

Now more than ever, hospitals are trying to find ways to keep their beds full. Look through your local newspaper and you will see ads for hospitals promoting themselves as the place for you to come. Hospitals are beginning to treat patients as consumers, and patients should approach hospitals as consumers as well.

Outpatient Procedures

Another way of saving money is to ask about having surgeries done as an outpatient. Many health insurance plans insist on surgery being performed in this manner. When you are an outpatient you arrive at the hospital early in the morning and go home later that same day. With some kinds of surgery this might work fine. Be sure you find out ahead of time, however, what care will be needed after you are released from the hospital. Will you need someone to drive you home? Should someone stay with you that night? What kind of reactions should you anticipate? What are potential postsurgical complications? If a complication arises, what should you do? Who should you call? Make sure you are given a phone number and the name of a medical professional to talk to. Do not accept being told to call the main hospital number and "anyone will be able to help you." If you don't think you will be able to take care of yourself and you don't have someone to help you out at home, make sure your doctor and the hospital staff are aware of this so arrangements can be made.

Since outpatient surgery is such an economical alternative to inpatient surgery, some doctors have taken to performing surgeries in their offices or at free-standing clinics. If you are considering these options, be aware that outpatient surgery is unregulated. There are no certification standards to be met. It is risky to have general anesthesia in a doctor's office, a free-standing clinic, or a dentist's office. If something should go wrong during the procedure, there would be no way to resuscitate you. You would need to be taken to the closest hospital emergency room, and that might take too long.

Cooperative Health Care

Ask if your hospital has a cooperative health-care program. In this kind of program, health-care workers teach patients about their illnesses, treatment, and recovery.

Family members are expected to take part in the care of the patient while he is in the hospital. In addition to saving up to a third of the cost of a normal hospital room, patients in these programs more easily make the transition from the hospital to home.

Even in traditional hospital settings, family members may be asked to take care of the patient themselves, and *not* be offered any savings. When this happens, ask what adjustment will be made to the bill. When I was in chemotherapy, my one-year-old daughter needed to have surgery. As my husband and I followed the nurse from the recovery room to our daughter's room, the nurse started explaining to us how to care for our child while she was in the hospital. She explained they just didn't have enough nurses and that this care would be our responsibility. My husband then explained that we were paying the hospital to have our daughter stay there to recuperate from surgery. The nurses would be responsible for her care, not us. We would be there a great deal of the time, but we were going to be keeping our daughter company, not acting as her nurses.

Don't let the nurses or anyone else at the hospital intimidate you. You are paying for the services they provide. If they are not happy with the situation, have them talk to your doctor. Let them know that you can always go to another hospital. As a health-care consumer, not only do you want to *save* money, you want to make sure that you receive the care you are paying for.

Emergency Rooms

Hospital emergency rooms are the most overused component of our health-care system. Two California researchers found that "unnecessary trips," that is, visits to the emergency room for treatment of nonemergency conditions such as hiccups or ingrown toenails, added between $5 billion and $7 billion to the country's medical bill in 1993.[3] If you use the emergency room this way, in addition to paying far more than you should for the services you receive, you won't always get quality care. If you are seriously ill or have had a severe injury, there is no better place to be than the emergency room. You will get the care you need. However, if you have a sore throat or are feeling tired, you will get better comprehensive care from your family doctor.

One of the main reasons people utilize emergency rooms for nonemergency problems is that they get sick when their doctor's office is closed or they don't have a doctor of their own. But there are other ways of dealing with these problems. If at three o'clock in the afternoon you suddenly feel sick, don't tell yourself you can wait until tomorrow to call the doctor. Call now! If on Friday morning you wake up with a bad sore throat, don't wait until it turns into something more serious before you call the doctor. Call now!

For those times when you get sick on a Saturday, late at night, or when you don't know where else to go, instead of heading down to your local hospital emergency room, investigate urgent-care centers in your area. Also referred to as "Doc in a Box," urgent-care centers are free-standing health-care centers that offer doctor as well as lab services. Although their hours vary, many are open from 8 A.M. to 8 P.M. Fees charged, although less than those of emergency rooms, are more than regular doctors' charges.

---

[3]"Unneeded ER Trips Cost Billions," *The Oregonian,* February 4, 1995, p. E2.

Most people choose the emergency room they go to on the basis of the hospital's reputation. But the care you receive in an emergency room may not always be the same quality as the care you would receive as an inpatient in that hospital. In an effort to cut back on expenses and make money, many hospitals contract out their emergency room work to independent companies. Be aware that these independent companies are not monitored by any state or federal agencies. Neither are they regulated by the American Medical Association. The hospitals in these situations act only as landlords, collecting rent each month from the renters. Check out the emergency room you plan to use in advance. Ask if it is run by the hospital or a separate medical entity.

Fees Are Negotiable

Medicine is a business and all business practices apply, including negotiation. Don't let the fact that you're dealing with highly trained medical professionals intimidate you into accepting prices that seem too high. If you feel you are not receiving value for the money you are spending, ask for lower prices or *find a new doctor.*

But remember—as in any other consumer issue, price is not the most important thing. Good quality at a fair price is what you want. Here are some ways you can save money:

- *Question excessive bills.* Maybe a mistake was made.

- *Don't pay for services not provided.* Look over your bills when you receive them. If you see charges for items or services you never received, have those charges removed. Many new mothers

of baby daughters have been surprised at
hospital bills that included charges for her
child's circumcision!

- *Rely on an internist or general practitioner as
  your primary physician.* Specialists charge more
  for office visits, and they will only be concerned
  with what pertains to their specialty. Of course, if
  your primary physician is stumped and doesn't
  know how to proceed, ask him to refer you to a
  specialist who would be able to help.

- *Investigate alternative health-care providers.*
  Doctors are not your only choice of health-care
  provider. Nurse-practitioners are registered nurses
  with master's degrees or other advanced training.
  They charge as much as 40 percent less than
  doctors and spend more time with their patients.[4]
  If you are pregnant you may want to consider
  seeing a certified nurse-midwife. These practitioners are licensed nurses with graduate degrees and
  national certification. You can save money while
  receiving quality care. Make sure you confirm the
  acceptability of these choices to your health
  insurance company—some companies may not
  cover these alternatives.

- *Newest doesn't mean best.* The newest test,
  treatment, or drug may not be any better for you
  than a current procedure, but the newest will
  always be more expensive.

---

[4]Jane Bennett Clark, "New Choices in Who Cares for You,"
Kiplinger's Personal Finance Magazine, November 1993, p. 124.

- *Open a health-care spending account at work.* More and more employers are offering their employees the opportunity to open health-care spending accounts. Employees designate a certain amount of money to be deducted from their paychecks *before* taxes and deposited in a special account. This money can be used to pay any out-of-pocket medical expenses—not insurance premiums, however, and any money left in the account at the end of the year is lost.

How to Question Insurance Company Decisions

There is a grave misconception among the general public that health insurance companies are always right, or, even when they're wrong, there's nothing to be done about it. Neither of those assumptions is true. If you feel you are not getting the coverage you've paid for, or if your health insurance company continually rejects claims for services you feel should be covered, question them.

Make sure you submit claims for drug expenditures. Insurance companies save a lot of money by not automatically paying pharmacies for prescriptions purchased. A large percentage of the public sees it as too much trouble to do the paperwork for only five to ten prescriptions a year. When you add up those out-of-pocket costs over the years, however, you'll find it worthwhile to get reimbursed.

Rejected Claims

Most insurance companies know that the general public will not question their decisions. Their attitude is that the average person does not know how or will not take the time to do what is necessary to have rejected charges reconsidered. This perception has also helped Medicare save a lot of money by rejecting many of the claims submitted.

Many Medicare claims are rejected as "medically unnecessary." High school graduates with *no medical training* make nine-tenths of the decisions on Medicare claims. So don't think that your insurance company "must know what they're doing" when they reject claims. The decisions may be haphazard. Challenge your health insurance company's decisions not to pay. Resubmit claims and demand an explanation of why the charges were not covered.

There are many reasons your claim may have been denied. If the company states that there is a lack of documentation, ask exactly what is needed, and send it. Save everything! If you haven't been doing this, do it from now on. Another reason a claim may be rejected is that the doctor's office submitted it with the wrong code. Call your doctor's office, have them check the code that was assigned, and if it was in error, have the claim resubmitted correctly.

It doesn't take much extra time to question why an insurance company is rejecting your claim. The money you save by not paying for things your insurance company should cover will make that time well worthwhile.

Negotiate, Negotiate, Negotiate!

If you call a doctor's office and ask the charge for an office visit, his staff will be the first to tell you "it depends." Yes, *it depends!* Do you have insurance? What kind of insurance? Do you *have* to see a doctor, or could a nurse-practitioner do the job? Other issues can be negotiated as well. For example, do you have twins, triplets, or more? Talk to your pediatrician about getting a discount on office visits.

Chapter 7

Women's Health Care

Health-care consumers know the importance of working closely with their doctors to get the care they need. Unfortunately, in the arena of women's health care, still more effort is necessary. Women must be extremely vigilant to ensure that their specific needs are being met. Read the medical literature and treatment protocols and investigate the procedures in which new drugs are tested, and you will see that most are based on results gathered from young *men*. It has commonly been assumed that treatments appropriate for men would work as well for women. The health-care community is finally coming to the realization that this is not true. This doesn't mean that substantial progress is being made in changing that assumption— it just means that doctors are *beginning* to understand that the accepted treatments and drugs may not be the best choices in dealing with women's health-care concerns.

Not only must women work closely with their doctors, they must make sure their doctors understand that the specific effectiveness for *women* of tests and treatments must be scrutinized.

Women make office visits to doctors twice as often as men, they undergo more outpatient surgery, and they are hospitalized more often. Most young women first see a gynecologist around age eighteen. From that point on, they will visit their doctor at least once a year. Some people question this annual schedule and think that it is merely a doctor's attempt to increase his fees. But there is sound reasoning behind annual checkups. Around age eighteen women have physically matured and are looking for independent sources of information on preventing pregnancy, infections, and diseases. They are also looking for confirmation that they are normal.

Gynecology

Chapter 2 suggested how to find the best doctor for you, but women should consider some additional things when choosing a gynecologist. In addition to checking credentials and researching the doctor's educational background, make sure that the doctor is someone you can trust: someone who has the ability to listen to your concerns and explain things so that you will understand.

Gynecologists have subspecialties as well, like obstetrics, infertility, and oncology. Be aware that not all gynecologists are obstetricians. Obstetricians are the doctors who are most often sued. Everyone wants a perfect baby, and when they don't have one, they blame the obstetrician. Doctors who don't want to worry about the constant threat of malpractice suits and want to avoid astronomically high malpractice insurance rates prefer to practice only gynecology. If your doctor is a gynecologist, and you plan on having children at some point, you will have to find an obstetrician later on.

Primary Care Physicians:
Internist–General Practitioner or OB-GYN?

You may wonder where an OB-GYN fits into your overall health-care needs. Many women think of their gynecologist as their only doctor. In some managed-care programs, gynecologists do act as primary care physicians, whereas other programs use them only as specialists. Check your health-care policy to see what your options are.

You may not be receiving complete health care if your OB-GYN is acting as your primary care physician. Gynecology and obstetrics are considered surgical specialties, even though in practice they primarily involve preventive care: Pap smears, birth control information, birth control prescriptions, and routine prenatal care. Internists and general practitioners are medical specialists. They are familiar with a wide range of health problems and may be the better choice to watch over *all* your health-care needs. Whereas gynecologists receive one year of training in general medicine, internists and general practitioners undergo over three years of training to become primary care doctors. They are aware of concerns that the OB-GYN may not consider.

You will also want to weigh carefully the choice of a family doctor or general practitioner in place of a gynecologist. OB-GYNs receive three years of training in obstetrics and gynecology, whereas family practitioners are required to take only one month of gynecology and two months of obstetrics training. OB-GYNs who were certified in or after 1986 must be tested every ten years in order to be recertified. Recertification ensures that the doctor is up to date on current procedures.

Make sure your health care is coordinated between your primary physician and your OB-GYN. See that both doctors receive test results and are aware of any medications you are taking. If your gynecologist is the only doctor you go to, make sure that he is apprised of that fact. The two of you will need to ensure that your preventive and primary health-care needs are being met.

Should Your OB-GYN Be a Woman?

When I was just out of college I began looking for a gynecologist. I asked my internist whom he would recommend and told him I preferred a woman doctor. My internist told me he could refer me to a woman doctor or the best OB-GYN he knew. I told him I wanted the name of the best doctor.

There is not much substantiated difference in the quality of care given by male and female OB-GYNs, although the demand for women gynecologists is high. This is easily understandable. Patients likely feel less embarrassed discussing extremely intimate issues with a woman. Women gynecologists are said to provide more preventive care, but I know that my male gynecologist has always emphasized prevention. Decide what is most important to you.

Your First Office Visit

Try to set up a get-acquainted appointment with the doctor before you need an examination. This will give you an opportunity to talk to the doctor fully dressed and preferably not in the examining room. Compatibility is the most important thing in this doctor-patient relationship. You must feel comfortable with your doctor.

Come prepared with a list of questions, your family's medical history, and your own reproductive history. Your personal reproductive history—number of kids, miscarriages, date of last menstrual period, birth control use, abortions, and sexually transmitted diseases—is very important, as well as your general health. During the interview, you'll want to ask how the doctor feels about mammograms, hysterectomies, and unnecessary surgery. Does she keep up to date with the latest findings and procedures? If you ask questions to which she doesn't know the answers, will she research the issues?

If you're uncomfortable going to the doctor by yourself, ask whether you can bring someone with you like your mom, husband, sister, or girlfriend. If the answer is no, ask why. The doctor may feel that it's easier for you to talk freely without the presence of a third person.

If you are uncomfortable with the questions your doctor asks, how he talks, or his demeanor, or if you feel something is just not right, leave and *find another doctor.*

Recently a lot of attention has been focused on gynecologists who sexually abuse their patients. In Portland, Oregon, in 1994, information came out about a doctor who was accused of molesting dozens of patients during a twenty-year period. Past patients of his said they had filed complaints against him, yet nothing had been done. When the media brought this situation to light, even more women came forward with additional allegations. Some of these women had been the doctor's patients for several years, others for just a few visits. He was well known, with a good reputation in the community.

What these women went through and what they learned from that experience can serve to educate you. This doctor talked in an obscene manner, used slang, and told dirty jokes. He never had a female nurse in the room when he did an exam. When he touched his patients inappropriately, the women thought something was wrong with *them;* the doctor couldn't *possibly* be doing what they thought he was doing.

Some of the women who were his patients now refuse to go to any doctor. It doesn't matter how sick they are, they would rather die than put their trust in another doctor. One woman I spoke with is pregnant with her first child. This is the *only* reason she now goes to a doctor, even though it's been two years since her experience. When she goes to an appointment, she brings her husband and her therapist with her. Her OB-GYN is a woman, and she says she will never go to a male doctor again. I asked this woman which she would choose if she had to decide between a woman doctor and the best doctor there is. She told me she would go to the woman doctor.

If there's a lesson to be learned here, it is to trust your feelings and your intuition. If you are not comfortable with a doctor, for *any* reason, leave!

Other questions you will want answered by the doctor or his office staff:

- Can he be reached by phone? How soon will he get back to you? The answers to these questions are extremely important when you're pregnant.

- Will he answer questions over the phone, or will you always have to make an appointment to come in? Some patients feel that unless a doctor will do most of his "doctoring" over the phone, he is just trying to drum up fees. This is not true. Some questions can be answered easily over the phone; drugs can sometimes be refilled over the phone. But if the doctor hasn't seen you in a year, and you want a prescription refilled, he'll want to see you to update your case. It is hard for a doctor to diagnose over the phone. He will want to make sure that he is not missing something, as he might if he took your word that "it's the same old thing."

- How far in advance is the doctor booked? Can you be "fit in" in an emergency?

- When your doctor is not available, is the doctor who covers for him a board-certified OB-GYN? This will be extremely important if you are pregnant, for your doctor may not be available when you're ready to deliver.

- Make sure the doctor is comfortable with a team relationship. If it makes him uncomfortable for you to ask questions, *find a new doctor.*

- What about the quality of the lab that is used to process Pap smears? A couple of years ago it turned out that some labs, to cut costs, employed medical students who took tests home with them to read. This practice is unacceptable. The quality of the test results is as important as the quality of the care you receive.

If you've been going to the same doctor for years but don't really know anything about him, you may want to start asking now, before you get pregnant or become seriously ill.

When it's time for your exam, again, ask questions. What will be done? Why? Will it hurt? How long will the appointment take? If you know what to expect, you will feel less apprehensive.

Whenever you call the doctor's office for an appointment, give the reason you are coming in. That way the staff will know how much time to schedule. If you need to talk

to the doctor about several things, let the staff know that
you will need some extra time for your appointment.

Obstetrics

So you're going to have a baby! The relationship between doctor and patient is extremely important during
pregnancy. Make sure you can talk to your doctor about
anything. It is vital that your doctor listen to you and help
you make the decisions *you* want to make. Is this an unexpected pregnancy? Will your doctor help you with your
options? Do the doctor's views match yours? Will they
color how he treats you and responds to your needs?
Is your doctor more interested in promoting his own
agenda?

There are a host of different options in childbirth
today. Is your doctor flexible or does he simply go by the
book regardless of what you personally may want?

Choices for Maternity Care

You have many choices when it comes to how you
bring your baby into this world. If you are dealing with an
uncomplicated pregnancy, you may want to consider a
certified nurse-midwife or lay midwife. If you are expecting problems, a medical doctor might be a better choice.
Research your options and their costs thoroughly, and
then make sure that you get what you want.

Obstetrician or Family Practitioner Most parents-to-
be insist that a physician be in attendance during pregnancy and delivery. If this is your choice, be sure to
ask about costs. Your obstetrician's office probably has
printed information on costs, required visits, and generally

everything you'll need to know. Is your doctor part of a group practice? Will you be seeing everyone in the practice? Most doctors' practices insist that you have at least one appointment with each of the doctors in the group during your pregnancy. That way, if your doctor is not on call when it is time for you to deliver your baby, you will have already met the doctor who is on call. Make sure your doctor knows about your wishes with regard to the delivery. Do you want your husband there? Do you want painkillers?

Certified Nurse-Midwife A certified nurse-midwife is a registered nurse who has completed at least one year of obstetric training in an approved graduate midwifery program, has demonstrated clinical experience, and has passed the American College of Nurse-Midwives national certification exam. Certified nurse-midwives have licenses or permits to practice in their home states, although Maine, Minnesota, Missouri, Oregon, and Virginia do not recognize or require certification. Different states have different restrictions on the functions certified nurse-midwives may perform.

A certified nurse-midwife deals with normal, uncomplicated pregnancies. If problems come up during the pregnancy she will refer you to a doctor. If you anticipate needing a doctor, investigate this possibility in advance. Ask your certified nurse-midwife which doctors she usually works with and see if they meet your expectations.

Lay Midwife You will find lay midwives delivering babies mostly in home settings. They are not licensed and they have no formal training in obstetrics. They usually practice in areas where medical care is not available. State laws governing lay midwives vary greatly.

Caesarian Sections

Caesarean deliveries in the United States make up approximately 22 percent of total births.[1] One question you should ask of *anyone* providing your maternity care is how they feel about the high incidence of Caesarean sections (C-sections). Most nonphysician providers will tell you that, should problems arise, they would call in a doctor. If this is not their standard procedure, ask how they do deal with complications.

In the past, most doctors felt that if a woman had had one C-section, all her subsequent deliveries should be by C-section as well. This has proved not to be necessary, but some doctors still insist on the practice. If you have had a C-section but would like to attempt a vaginal delivery, make sure the doctor you choose will work with you to accomplish this. If he has reservations about it, *find a new doctor.*

When a woman I knew had her three children, each time her doctor told her what day and time she was to check into the hospital. Either this man was extremely psychic or he didn't want to have to work on his days off. Even for her first delivery, when a C-section was not expected, the doctor prescheduled her delivery time. Things have changed in the past forty-five years, however. Deliveries usually are no longer scheduled just for the convenience of the doctor. C-sections are complicated surgeries that require recuperation time, made more difficult by having a newborn to take care of. They should not be performed haphazardly.

---

[1]Stephanie Young, "New Research on C-Section Rates," *Glamour,* February 1995, p. 42.

Another reason doctors do C-sections is to protect themselves. Everyone wants to have a perfect baby. When they don't, they are ready to sue the doctor, the hospital, and everyone else they perceive responsible. Unfortunately, not all babies are born perfect. Doctors sometimes try to avoid potential lawsuits by second-guessing themselves and performing a large number of C-sections. Investigate the C-section statistics of your doctor and of the hospital where you will deliver. *Now* is the time to get answers to any questions you may have. Ask under what circumstances your doctor would perform a C-section. If you are not satisfied with the answer, *find a new doctor.*

Where to Have Your Baby

Just as you have many choices as to who will care for you during your pregnancy, you have many choices of where to go to have your baby.

Hospital Hospitals are the most common choice of place to deliver babies. Most doctors insist on using a hospital. Although most deliveries will be uncomplicated, should problems arise, the hospital is the place to be. It has the necessary equipment and its staff will know how to deal with whatever comes up. You may have to give up some freedom of choice, however. Hospitals have standard procedures for childbirth. These may include IVs, enemas, fetal monitoring, episiotomies, epidurals, induced labor, and use of forceps. Do you feel comfortable with these procedures? Discuss your wishes with your doctor or health-care professional and agree on what will and will not be done. Make sure the hospital is aware of and will follow through on your wishes.

Managed care is changing a great deal about hospital care during and after childbirth. The most profound change is the length of the hospital stay. Most health-care plans allow a twenty-four- to thirty-six-hour stay for routine deliveries and three days for Caesarean births. If you don't think this is sufficient time for your specific situation, make sure your doctor is willing to do battle with your insurance company and will not just send you home, unable to care for yourself or your baby. However, you may want to leave the hospital as soon as possible and recuperate in the comfort of your own home. Make sure your doctor will listen to your wishes. If you want to leave the hospital early, talk to your doctor and have him confirm that you and your baby can be discharged. As doctors will be the first to tell you, the hospital is no place for a healthy woman and baby!

Birth Center or Women's Center A birth center or women's center is a free-standing facility not affiliated with a hospital. The philosophy of such facilities is that childbirth is a natural process not requiring medical intervention. If you are looking for this approach, that is fine, but be aware that there is usually no doctor on the premises should medical help be necessary.

Home Birth You may want to have your baby at home. If you live in a rural community far from any hospital or birth center, you may have no other options. It is important to discuss this choice with your health-care provider. Make sure she is comfortable delivering a baby in a home setting. If she is not, *find a new doctor.*

When you are pregnant, everyone you know will be telling you what they did, what *their* doctor told *them,* and what *you* should be doing. Assure them that you have faith in your doctor and that you and she are doing what is best for you and the baby.

Specific Concerns for Women

The exclusion of women from most clinical tests and trials dictates that all women should be cautious when considering any treatment, procedure, or drug recommended by doctors. The reasons for excluding women from tests and trials may seem to make sense: fear that experimental drugs and treatments might harm the reproductive capabilities of women involved in the studies; concern that women's menstrual cycles might skew test results by affecting the way drugs are metabolized; or the assumption that illnesses and the drugs to treat them would affect both men and women the same. But this assumption doesn't make sense; we don't know how these drugs or treatments will affect women. Many drugs and treatments that are currently being prescribed were tested only on men.

Doctors will tell you that taking aspirin daily will help prevent heart attacks. But that knowledge was gained from a study of 22,000 *male* doctors. It is not known if the same protective effect works on women. The following sections discuss some other health issues that concern women.

Birth Control

A woman's birth control needs will change many times during her lifetime. In their twenties most women want to prevent pregnancy while protecting their fertility. During this period, the Pill is the most popular contraceptive choice. It is reliable as well as reversible.

Not all women will be able to take the Pill. In the past, the only other choices were diaphragms, spermicides, IUDs, cervical caps, or contraceptive sponges. Now two other long-term methods can be considered—Norplant and Depo-Provera.

Norplant is a long-lasting (five years) contraceptive method. Six narrow inch-long rods containing synthetic hormones are implanted into the upper arm. As with every other birth control option, there are side effects to consider, including irregular bleeding and weight gain. Controversy surrounds the use of Norplant, and it is expensive: Clinics and doctors pay $365, and patients are sometimes charged more than $500, for the rods with an insertion kit. In other countries Norplant costs clinics as little as $23, without the kit. Talk to your doctor about this. Negotiate the cost with her, and ask her to negotiate with the drug company she buys it from. It is important to remember that if you choose to use Norplant, it does nothing to protect you from sexually transmitted diseases.

Depo-Provera is administered by a shot of synthetic hormones that lasts for three months. It is convenient and dependable, and does not cause nausea; breast tenderness is a side effect. Since this is a relatively new option, little is known about long-term effects. Like Norplant, Depo-Provera does not protect against sexually transmitted diseases.

In their mid-thirties and forties, many American women have completed their families. They begin thinking of sterilization—either vasectomies for their partners or tubal ligations for themselves—as their contraceptive choice. Although doctors will tell you that these procedures can be reversed, they should be thought of as permanent. Did you know that although many insurance companies will pay for sterilization, they won't reimburse a dime for having it reversed? Sterilization will prevent unplanned pregnancies, but you will still have to protect yourself from sexually transmitted diseases.

Unplanned pregnancy is as big a problem for women in their forties as it is for teenagers. This may be explained by the fact that as women get closer to menopause, their cycles become irregular and they begin to feel they are too old to get pregnant.

Talk to your doctor and ask what she thinks would be the best method for you to consider, whatever your age. You'll need to discuss your lifestyle so you can make an informed choice. Are you married? Are you breast-feeding? Do you have a medical problem that may make a particular method unworkable? For instance, women who have migraine headaches should not use the Pill. New methods are always coming out—for example, the female condom and the morning-after pill. You and your doctor, evaluating these choices together, will be able to reach a decision suited to you.

Infertility

Just as birth control is an important issue for young women, infertility has become important to women as they get older. After years of trying to make sure they didn't get pregnant, many women in their thirties and forties are finding that it isn't as easy to conceive as they had expected.

If this is one of your concerns, talk to your doctor. Can he treat this problem? Should you see a specialist? What procedures does your doctor suggest? How aggressive do you and your doctor want to be? What factors would your decision be based on: cost, time required, or success rate of a particular method?

Infertility has become a big-money business. In 1994 Americans spent $2 billion trying to get pregnant. There are no guarantees in this process, and it is important to realize what you are getting into. Make sure you are dealing with a doctor you can trust.

At one of my seminars, I spoke with a woman in her late twenties. She and her husband had just decided to start their family. She had gone to her gynecologist and asked him if she should be doing anything special to prepare for getting pregnant. Her doctor told her that she would probably not be able to get pregnant easily, since she was "older," so she should proceed as though she were infertile. The doctor explained all the new procedures available to infertile women. This woman went home, discussed the situation with her husband, and then found a new doctor. She delivered a healthy baby boy one year later, with no intervention needed.

Wanting children is a very emotional thing. Some doctors may play on your fears to force unneeded medical procedures on you. Act like the health-care consumer you are. Research your doctor thoroughly. If he starts insisting on invasive and expensive procedures, question him. Are these necessary now or just options to consider in the future? What percentage of your doctor's practice are infertility patients? Does he treat all his patients as though they were infertile even if they're not? Make sure you are satisfied with the answers you receive. If you're not, *find a new doctor.*

If you find that infertility *is* a problem for you, talk to your doctor about your options. Let your doctor know what you are comfortable doing. Will drugs like Clomid or Pergonal help, or will they cause other problems? What are the side effects? Fertility drugs have been in use for a relatively short time, and it is not known what all the long-term health effects will be. A study from the Pacific Fertility Center in San Francisco found that prolonged use of Clomid may actually *reduce* the chance of conceiving.[2] Researchers at the University of Washington and the Fred Hutchinson Cancer Research Center have found that women who were treated for at least a year with infertility drugs have a two and a half times greater risk of ovarian cancer than do untreated infertile women.[3] If these drugs don't work or are not safe, what other choices are there? In vitro fertilization (IVF)?

Many couples see IVF as the answer to their infertility problems. But of all couples undergoing the procedure, an average of only 17 percent end up with a baby.[4] Ask your doctor if IVF is an option you should consider. Health insurance *will not cover* many infertility procedures. Read through your policy and learn what is covered and what is not. If you believe the company rejects claims when they shouldn't, question it. It's important that you discuss this with your doctor. Your husband should also be included in these discussions.

In addition to working with a good doctor, research any fertility clinic you deal with. There are more than three hundred fertility clinics in the United States. Before going to one, ask to see their success statistics and proof of their accreditation. Overall, fertility clinics have a 25 percent success rate.[5]

Did you know that even if you have a child you could still have a problem getting pregnant again? This is called secondary infertility and is experienced by one in six couples who try to get pregnant. As with any other situation,

---

[2]"A Common Fertility Drug Might Backfire," *Self,* September 1994, p. 59.

[3]Margot Slade, "Managing Menopause," *American Health,* December 1994, p. 6.

[4]"The Baby Chase," *U.S. News and World Report,* December 5, 1994, pp. 86–94.

[5]"The Baby Chase," *U.S. News and World Report,* December 5, 1994, pp. 84–94.

talk to your doctor and discuss your options. The health-care consumer realizes that the best choice is an informed choice.

Hormone Replacement Therapy

All women have to deal with menopause as they get older. Did you know that women are more likely to learn about menopause from television talk shows than from their own doctors? It's great that they're learning about it, but, as with all other medical issues, each person's needs are different. You can listen to or read about how other women are making their choices, but their decisions should not necessarily be yours.

Everyone has different views on the use of hormone replacement therapy. Discuss your concerns with your doctor. Ask about the benefits, the risks, and the other options that are open to you. The February 1995 issue of *Prevention* magazine discussed diet therapy as a way of dealing with menopause. Because this is a new concept, your doctor may not have heard of it yet. Ask him to question his peers and see if diet therapy may be of benefit to you.

Women whose hair goes gray before age forty are four times more likely than average to develop osteoporosis.

Treating menopause is a personal choice and must meet your specific needs. Many women will tell you that menopause is a natural process and you should just accept all its effects. Your situation, however, may be different. Ask your doctor how hormone replacement therapy helps prevent heart disease, cancer, and osteoporosis. Women whose hair goes gray before age forty are four times more likely than average to develop osteoporosis.[6] What are

---

[6]Jane Shiyen Chou, "Osteoporosis Warning Sign," *Family Circle,* March 14, 1995, p. 53.

your risks, hereditary or otherwise? Talk to your doctor
and come to the decision that works best for you.

Hysterectomy

If your doctor suggests that you should have a hysterectomy, ask why. Hysterectomies are said to be the unnecessary surgery most often performed on women, and
no one should allow one without getting a second, third,
or even fourth opinion. Ask your doctor why she feels *you*
need to have this surgery. Some doctors feel that after a
woman has had all the children she wants there is no reason for her *not* to have a hysterectomy. Is that why the
doctor wants *you* to have one? This may be considered
unnecessary surgery.

There are viable medical reasons for hysterectomies.
Surgery would be considered necessary in cases of invasive cancer, severe infection, uncontrollable bleeding,
and some complications of childbirth. But beware if
the reasons being given for surgery are vaginal discharge, backache, hormonal imbalance, or permanent
birth control. There are other, *better* ways of solving
these problems.

Find out *why* a hysterectomy is being recommended.
Research your options and make your wishes known. A
study in the *American Journal of Public Health* as reported
in the February 1995 issue of *Self* magazine found that patients of recently trained gynecologists who voiced reservations about the surgery were often spared unnecessary
hysterectomies.[7]

---

[7]"Older Male Gynecologists Most Likely to Perform Hysterectomies," *Self,* February 1995, p. 75.

Heart Disease, Stroke, Lung Cancer, and Breast Cancer

There are some diseases that people don't think about when it comes to women's health: heart disease, stroke, and lung cancer are three of these. Also, some might think of breast cancer as *only* a woman's disease, but that is not the case. According to the American Cancer Society, in the United States approximately 1,000 men a year are diagnosed with breast cancer. All of these diseases are of special concern to women.

Heart Disease The feature article in the February 1995 issue of *Reader's Digest* was "Is Your Husband Headed for a HEART ATTACK?" The article is condensed from "What's Your Heart Attack Risk?" which appeared in the October 1994 issue of *Consumer Reports on Health*. The article includes a test for men and women listing risk factors for heart attacks. Each risk factor is characterized as increasing women's chances of having a heart attack more than men's. Yet *Reader's Digest* chose to title its article "Is Your Husband Headed for a HEART ATTACK?" This is a not-so-subtle example of the pervasive bias against women's health care.

Heart disease is the number one killer of women, as well as of men, in the United States.[8] Heart disease usually goes undetected and untreated in women. One of the reasons is that the warning signs women experience may not

---

[8]*Heart and Stroke Facts: 1995 Statistical Supplement,* American Heart Association pamphlet.

be the same as the signs exhibited in men. Doctors say that some of the symptoms women display are

- Vague abdominal discomfort
- Nausea, and vomiting
- Fatigue
- Shortness of breath
- Arm and/or chest pain[9]

It has been thought that women were hormonally protected from heart disease until after menopause. If a premenopausal woman had symptoms that suggested heart disease, doctors tended to ignore it. The woman passed it off as a pulled muscle, stress, or indigestion, or just ignored it too. But such symptoms can't be ignored. Thirty percent of women between thirty-five and sixty-four who suffer heart attacks die within a year. Only 16 percent of men in that same age group die.[10]

The American Medical Women's Association recently announced a three-year educational program for doctors to focus on cardiac disease in women.[11] This is a much-needed step in the right direction.

Stroke Stroke is the nation's third leading cause of death, after heart attack and cancer.[12] On average, someone

---

[9]"A Woman's Heart," *Ladies' Home Journal,* October 1994, pp. 112–118.

[10]*Heart and Stroke Facts: 1995 Statistical Supplement,* American Heart Association pamphlet.

[11]Beth Weinhouse, "The Ways of a Woman's Heart," *New Woman,* February 1995, p. 48.

[12]"Gail McBride, "Stroke—A Prevention and Survival Kit," *American Health,* January/February 1995, p. 64.

suffers a stroke in the United States every minute; every three and a half minutes someone dies of one. More men than women have a stroke, yet sixty-one percent of those who die from strokes are women.[13]

Lung Cancer   Cancer is the number two killer of women. Lung cancer is the leading cause of cancer death, followed by breast cancer.[14] Lung cancer rates have been increasing because of the greater incidence of women smoking, and in a recent study, female smokers were found to have twice the chance of contracting lung cancer as males. At this time there seems to be no explanation for this disparity. Most of the participants in the study smoked about a pack a day and had smoked for about forty years.[15] In addition to using our consumer skills to receive the quality care we require, women also need to use these skills to *prevent* illnesses when we can.

Breast Cancer   An estimated 207,000 women will be diagnosed with breast cancer this year.[16] The National Cancer Institute estimates that one out of eight women

---

[13]*Heart and Stroke Facts: 1995 Statistical Supplement,* American Heart Association pamphlet.

[14]*Cancer Facts and Figures—1995,* American Cancer Society pamphlet.

[15]H.A. Risch, G.R. Howe, M. Jain, J.D. Burch, E.J. Holowaty, and A.B. Miller, "Are Female Smokers at Higher Risk for Lung Cancer Than Male Smokers? A Case Control Analysis by Histologic Type." *American Journal of Epidemiology* (1993), issue 138, pp. 281–293.

[16]Rita Baron-Faust, with the physicians of the NYU Medical Center Women's Health Service and the Kaplan Comprehensive Cancer Center, *Breast Cancer: What Every Woman Should Know,* 1995, New York: William Morrow & Co.

will develop breast cancer in her lifetime. Evidence shows that early detection of breast cancer can save lives. Talk to your doctor about breast self-examination, how to do it, and when to do it. There is controversy around when and how often mammograms should be given. Discuss this issue with your doctor and you keep to the schedule you agree on. If your doctor seems reluctant to refer you for a mammogram, call him on it. Do you have risk factors he may not be considering? Have you felt a lump in your breast but your doctor wants you to just "wait and see?" Tell your doctor that you won't wait—your *life* depends on having this exam. If your doctor still wants to wait, *find a new doctor.*

Have your mammogram done only at a facility that has been certified by the Food and Drug Administration. This will assure you that trained technicians and modern equipment are being used. It is important to understand that a diagnosis of breast cancer does not mean that you're going to die from breast cancer. With early detection the chance of successful treatment is good.

Many of these diseases will not wait until you're older to strike. That is why it is so important to be a good health-care consumer. Be assertive; demand the care and information you need. You know your body better than anyone else. Don't let someone tell you that "it's all in your head" or that it's "just stress" when you know it's not. No one wants their headstone to read, "I told you I was sick!"

Chapter 8

Men's Health Care

The men I know are not used to approaching doctors assertively. If it were up to them, they probably wouldn't see doctors at all. Many men perceive being sick and going to doctors as signs of weakness of character. A medical appointment is not only an inconvenience but an admission to the world that the man is a failure because he hasn't avoided getting sick. But men *can*—and *do*—avoid going to the doctor.

If you ask most men why they finally went to the doctor, they will tell you it's because their mother, sister, significant other, or wife insisted on it and made the appointment for them. Let's stop this habit. Men need to take control of their own health-care needs. I don't think that is impossible. Men seem to apply the perception of sickness as some kind of character flaw only to themselves. When my daughter catches a cold, my husband is the first one on the phone to her doctor. If I consider rescheduling my doctor's appointment because I'm too busy, my husband will insist that I not put it off. But if he gets the flu and is still coughing four months later, he'll refuse to go to a doctor because "it'll go away by itself."

You would never want your car to run out of gas or break down on an empty road somewhere. You're going to make sure that the oil is changed regularly, that the proper quality of gas is used, and that the car is not driven too fast, too hard, or in hazardous conditions. You should be as devoted to the care of your body as you are to that of your car.

"I Don't Have Time to Be Sick"

When my husband gets a cold or the flu, his first response is, "I don't have time to be sick." Of course illness never waits around for the most convenient time to strike. But bad health doesn't just *happen* to us. Much of your health is within your control. Preventive care, such as eating well, exercising, getting enough sleep, and seeing your doctor for checkups will help you avoid bad health surprises.

The way you handle illness when it does occur can determine how long it will affect you. A thirty-something man in one of my seminars explained why he chose to "keep on going" when he got sick: "I can't call in sick with just a cold. I have to tough it out. Now, if the cold turns into bronchitis or pneumonia, I can stay home for at least a week, because *then* I'd be *sick!*"

When this man goes to work with his cold, he is infecting other people. They go home and infect their families, who go to *their* jobs and infect everyone there. If this man stayed home for a day or two when his cold was just a cold, think of all the lost work hours that would be saved. Men should think about their health-care needs in a logical manner—the same way they would approach a business transaction. When you don't feel well, go to the doctor. If the doctor can't work together with you to get you better, find out why not. And then find out what your next move should be.

The Differences Between Men's and Women's Health-Care Experiences

Men and women have very different experiences with doctors. Whereas women commonly go to the doctor for yearly checkups and examinations, men's visits to doctors usually take place under duress: when they're irritable and in pain. Because of this, men and women often have very different attitudes toward doctors.

Because of their experience with monthly menstruation, most women are well attuned to the workings of their bodies. They know from experience what is routine and acceptable and what is unusual and warrants a doctor's appointment. Going to the doctor is not a scary experience for most women because they are accustomed to going regularly.

Men, on the other hand, tend to go to the doctor only when something is very wrong. Thus when they visit the doctor they frequently get bad news, which makes them less inclined to return. Although they might have realized something was wrong weeks earlier, many men will put off a doctor's appointment because they don't want to hear that bad news. If men would go to the doctor when they first became aware of something unusual, their problems would be resolved early and would not become serious health threats.

As reported in the *Wall Street Journal,* many men are terrible patients, especially when their doctors are also men.[1] Researchers at the Health Institute of the New

---

[1]Ron Winslow, "Health Care" column, *Wall Street Journal,* July 9, 1993.

England Medical Center in Boston discovered that men were passive with a male doctor. They asked few questions and talked little about their symptoms. When dealing with women doctors, by comparison, men gave more than twice as much information regarding their condition. Since good communication between patient and doctor can contribute positively to a patient's health, most men are at a disadvantage. So what should they do?

Don't Delay Treatment

I'm not suggesting that you run to your doctor for every sniffle, cough, ache, or twinge. You wouldn't do that anyway. But be aware of your general health. If you've had a cold for a month and it keeps getting worse, maybe you should have it checked out. If you strain your back in a game of basketball and the next morning you can't get out of bed, call your doctor. Any health-care problem that doesn't get better with time needs to be discussed with your doctor.

Is It Really Only Stress?

Stress is the disease of the nineties. There is too much to do and not enough time: work and family obligations and all the emergencies that pop up in between. You may find yourself bothered by headaches, fatigue, sleeplessness, chest pains, shortness of breath, and anxiety, along with countless other symptoms.

When you finally go to the doctor, the diagnosis is "stress." You are told to take it easy, don't work so hard, find a hobby, take a vacation. You thank the doctor for his help and leave the office knowing you won't follow his advice. After all, it's nothing serious, just stress.

But stress *is* serious. Not only does it cause countless troublesome symptoms, it also weakens the immune system, leaving you vulnerable to many opportunistic infections and diseases. So don't just walk out of the office and ignore the doctor's advice. If you can't cut back on work or take that vacation, ask your doctor to recommend things you *can* do.

Be aware too, however, that not everything is caused by stress. When you go to the doctor with a health problem, does he ask how your family life is? Is he always wondering if you are worried about something? If you feel your doctor tends to blame your symptoms on stress instead of exploring your concerns further, talk to him about it. Let your doctor know that you aren't asking him to do every test in the book, but you don't want your concerns to be automatically dismissed as stress.

Doing What
Your Doctor Says

The number one complaint doctors have about their male patients is noncompliance; they don't follow the prescribed treatment. If you're guilty of noncompliance, ask yourself why you're not doing what the doctor recommended. Did he give you a prescription that needs to be taken four times a day, and you just can't do that? Did he prescribe a medicine that makes you feel worse than the condition it's supposed to cure? Let your doctor know. Many choices are available among prescription medicines. Make sure your doctor realizes that getting well is important to you but that you need a plan you can follow. The doctor won't know what choices to make unless you discuss your requirements with him.

Specific Concerns for Men

Specific diseases and problems occur commonly in men. Discuss your personal habits and your family's medical history with your doctor. Many men like to feel they are invulnerable and continue to indulge in behavior that affects their well-being. Smoking, drinking, and bad eating habits can have a negative impact on anyone's general health. Make sure your doctor is aware of your "bad habits" so they can be considered in discussions of your health care.

Many men say they don't go to the doctor when they need to because they are afraid of being scolded about their habits. The doctor-patient relationship is different from an adult-child relationship. You should not be afraid of how a doctor will react to your habits. But you also need to be realistic. The doctor would be shirking her responsibility if she did not discuss with you the consequences of your actions. These discussions are handled in the context of preventive care and how you can improve your well-being. If you choose not to change your lifestyle, that's your business. But don't blame your doctor for discussing it. Helping you improve your health is her job.

Heart Attack

About one of every four people who die suddenly of a heart attack had no previous symptoms of heart disease.[2] What most likely brings on heart attacks is exposure to

---

[2]*Mayo Clinic® Family Health Book,* 1993, Eagan, Minn.: IVI Publishing, p. 15.

certain risk factors: High blood pressure, smoking, diabetes, and high-fat diets contribute to heart disease. Take control of your health care and do what is necessary to avoid preventable disease.

Stroke

Stroke is the third leading killer and a major cause of disability in the United States. Stroke will affect up to 30 percent more men than women. One third of the strokes in men occur before age sixty-five. In 1992, approximately 15,000 men under forty-five had strokes.[3] The good news is that strokes are preventable, but you need to start prevention strategies *now!* Discuss with your doctor what it takes to lessen your risk of stroke. Many doctors suggest that men lower their blood pressure, exercise, and stop smoking. Discuss with your own doctor what changes you should make in your lifestyle.

Prostate Cancer

Read the newspaper, watch television, or talk to friends and family and you will hear about prostate cancer. Prostate cancer is third among the types of cancer that kill American men. It is found mostly in individuals aged sixty to eighty and is more common in black men than in white men.[4] If it's detected early, prostate cancer can be cured, although once the symptoms begin to appear, a cure is less likely.

---

[3]*Heart and Stroke Facts: 1995 Statistical Supplement,* American Heart Association pamphlet.
[4]*Mayo Clinic® Family Health Book,* 1993, Eagan, Minn.: IVI Publishing, p. 5.

Researchers at the Memorial Sloan-Kettering Cancer Center found that abstaining from sex for a week before a prostate-cancer blood screening may give your doctor more accurate test results. Talk to your doctor about this if he suggests that you have this blood screen done.

If you should be diagnosed with prostate cancer, treatments are available. Now, in addition to surgery or being told to "wait and see," drugs are being used as treatment.

Testicular Cancer

Testicular cancer is usually detected in males between the ages of fifteen and thirty-five. It is more common in white men than in black men. If a man had one or both testicles undescended at birth, the risk of this cancer is greater. Testicular cancer can often be cured if it is detected and treated early. Call your doctor if you are concerned about this and discuss what you need to do.

Male Menopause

No one really agrees on the concept of "male menopause." Those who believe it exists state that men change as they grow older, just like women. Men begin to have physical problems due to aging, and that causes emotional problems. Male menopause is seen more as a psychological problem than a hormonal one.

If you think this condition may be affecting you or someone you know, talk to your doctor. Discuss your concerns and apprehensions. Do you need to talk to someone else about what's happening to you? Work with your doctor to ensure that you receive the health care and counseling you need.

Other Health-Care Concerns for Men

One of the particular dangers facing men in the health-care arena is that delayed treatment means advanced disease. This is a significant problem with diseases that have few or no symptoms. High blood pressure, high blood cholesterol, diabetes, and lung cancer are all health conditions made more difficult to treat because when they are found, it is usually after they have already caused serious health problems.

More than three million American men—half with diabetes—have elevated blood sugar and don't know it. This is particularly dangerous because men with diabetes are two to four times more likely than those without the disease to die from heart disease and six times more prone to suffer a stroke.[5] What can you do? Know what your health risks are. Did your parents or grandparents have chronic illnesses? You may be more susceptible to those same diseases. Discuss your family health history with your doctor and find out what you need to do to ensure your continued good health.

Preventive Health Care for Men

One of the reasons doctors prefer men to come in for regular checkups instead of waiting until something is wrong is that serious problems caught early have a far greater chance of being cured. Ask your doctor how often she thinks checkups are necessary, and check with your health insurance company to see if these visits are covered.

---

[5]"Men and Diabetes," *Men's Health,* September 1993, p. 33.

If your health insurance coverage does not include regular checkups, ask the company why not. Most health insurance companies cover yearly examinations and tests for women. Men's health care is as important as women's and should not be covered differently. Act like the health-care consumer you are and get what you need from your doctor and the health-care community.

Chapter 9

Senior Health Care

Caution: Skipping this chapter may endanger your health and the health of your family!

Senior health care is important to everyone. If it is not an element of your life in some way now, it will be. It is affecting your parents, your grandparents, and millions of others every day. The fastest-growing age group in the United States is people seventy-five years old and over. Like all other health-care consumers, seniors need to stand up for their needs and not allow others to intimidate them.

Preconceived Ideas About Seniors

When it comes to the subject of aging, preconceived ideas—both the doctor's and the patient's—can be harmful. The elderly population today is much different from what it was fifty years ago. For one thing, its members are a lot older. It is not unusual today for people to live to be eighty-five or older. At one time, the term "senior citizen" referred to anyone over fifty. Those who did not die while still working had little to do in retirement except sit and watch the world go by.

Today's senior citizens spend almost as many years in retirement as they did on the job. Sitting has been replaced by traveling, going back to school, playing tennis and golf, long-distance running, and bringing up grand-children. This state of affairs has led to the often-heard

123

comment, "If I'd known I was going to live this long, I'd have taken better care of myself."

Despite the recent changes, seniors still have to fight stereotypes. They are perceived as less flexible and less capable of learning than younger people. If they forget something, they're "getting senile"; if they become angry, they're "being crotchety." An assertive senior is seen as a problem to be managed. Perception becomes important here.

The biggest decline in memory skills happens in your thirties and forties. Very little memory loss takes place after fifty.

The biggest decline in memory skills happens in your thirties and forties. Very little memory loss takes place after fifty. What is being forgotten? A woman forgets to pick up her cleaning but remembers that next Thursday her favorite movie is on television. "Forgetting" may simply be a case of selective memory, with the emphasis on what is important to the individual.

Memory tests have compared seniors with younger people. Unfortunately, the tests were written and given by younger people, who look for what is lost with age and not what is gained. It may take a senior relatively longer to come up with an answer, but she has a lot more information to sift through.

Medical Mistreatment of the Elderly

In the American medical community there is a clear bias against older people. Doctors are not routinely taught geriatric medicine in medical school. In fact, only eight of the country's medical schools require separate courses in geriatric medicine, whereas *all* medical schools require courses in pediatrics and obstetrics.

There are about four thousand geriatrics specialists in this country, but as an older person you don't need one for routine care. You need a doctor who will listen to you and answer your questions completely. You need a doctor who will work with you to see that you get the health care you need. Most of all, remember that you have a unique perspective on what is happening in your own body.

Getting Older or Getting Sick

An 85-year-old woman I knew went to her doctor with some concerns: She had no energy, she had to nap in the afternoon, and she was always very cold. The doctor said, "You know, as we get older we start having some problems." The woman responded, "I've been getting older for the past 85 years; these problems just started two weeks ago."

It is simply not true that problems arise because "that's what happens when you get older." Forgetting is a perfect example. In the aging process, forgetting is not natural at sixty but may begin to occur after eighty. So if you're seventy-five and you can't remember, this may have more to do with a bad reaction to medicine or poor nutrition than with your age. Talk to your doctor. Tell him about your concerns and ask him what you can do to remedy the situation.

Believing health problems are age related rather than due to illness is the number one reason seniors don't go to doctors. They may have trouble walking; they may not hear well; their eyesight may be blurred. When they discuss these problems with friends and family they may be told, "These things happen." Don't believe it! Go to the doctor, tell him your symptoms, how long you've had them, and whether they're getting worse. Let the doctor evaluate the situation. Symptoms seniors experience may be out of the ordinary. Instead of crushing chest pain signaling a heart attack, they may feel fatigue.

It's also important *how* you tell your doctor about your symptoms. If every time you see the doctor you say you're tired, he may start ignoring your concern. If you have not been regularly complaining about such a problem but on one visit tell him you have been so tired you couldn't get out of bed, he will realize that this is not a routine complaint.

The fact that people are taking better care of themselves also makes a difference in distinguishing between what is age related and what is illness related. Starting back in 1968, there was an unexpected drop in mortality attributable to heart disease. The change was not due to medical intervention but to lifestyle changes: healthy diet, exercise, and quitting smoking. People had started taking care of themselves to prevent illness.

But no matter how well you take care of yourself, you *are* more apt to get sick as you get older. Those over 65 see a doctor at least seven to eight times a year because of illness, take twice as much medicine as all other age groups combined, and use 31.3 percent of all short hospital stays.[1]

A significant issue for seniors is depression. Major traumas are attached to getting older, and they have a big impact on health. One major problem is the loss of personal freedom and becoming dependent on others. Seniors may no longer be able to drive. Problems may develop in their relations with their middle-aged children. All of these things impact senior health care.

Undertreatment and Overtreatment

Since seniors use so much health care, you would think that doctors must have a great deal of information about how to treat them. This is not the case. Not much is

---

[1]U.S. Senate Special Committee on Aging, 1993, *Developments in Aging,* Washington, D.C.: U.S. Government Printing Office.

known about how seniors react to illness or respond to treatment. Those over 65 are routinely omitted from clinical trials and studies. The treatment plans and screening procedures for various illnesses are based on information gathered from healthy, young males.

As a result, treatment of elderly people is generally inadequate. They are not given tests when needed, they are given too many or not enough prescriptions, and surgeons either push surgery or refuse to do it. Seniors need to ask about the treatment options available and question the doctor about why she has chosen a specific treatment plan.

Even when properly diagnosed, seniors don't always get the care they need. Cancer patients over seventy-five are less likely to be offered radiation and chemotherapy than younger patients. Although heart disease is the leading killer of the elderly, seniors are less likely to receive medicines that reduce heart attack death rates. When disease is diagnosed, they are treated less aggressively.

Another problem in senior health care is *over* treatment. Multiple medications and conflicting therapies prescribed by different doctors can cause new problems because no one is overseeing the care being provided as a whole. You can prevent some problems by bringing all your prescriptions with you when you go to a new doctor. Show her all your medications, including OTC drugs, so she knows the types and dosages.

Some Problems with Drugs

Prescription and over-the-counter drugs are a great concern for seniors. A Harvard Medical School study found that the wrong drugs are given to one in four elderly patients.[2]

---

[2]*New York Times,* July 27, 1994, p. B7.

Prescribing the proper dosage is a concern as well. Many doctors don't realize that a correct dosage for a forty-five-year-old may be an overdose for a sixty-year-old. Seniors need smaller drug dosages because their metabolisms are slower. Studies in this area are limited; the effects of drugs on the elderly have only been tested in the last few years. Even when drugs are being properly monitored, prescription drugs can cause problems. Sedative use is a great concern in the elderly.

People over sixty-five make up 13 percent of the American population, yet they take 30 percent of all prescription drugs sold in this country.[3] A combination of drugs can create problems, but side effects from one drug often cause a doctor to prescribe another. It would be better to find an alternate first drug. As mentioned above, metabolism slows as we get older. Seniors need to be aware of this because medicines will build up in the system and eventually reach higher levels in the bloodstream than they should.

There are additional problems. In seniors, drug reactions sometimes aren't as expected. Instead of making the patient tired, a drug may make her nervous and agitated. The doctor may then prescribe a higher dose, thinking that the patient is not getting enough of the drug.

Although seniors are more prone to drug side effects, they are less likely to blame medicines than those aged forty to fifty. They aren't told often enough that the drug could cause problems, and they are therefore more likely to blame their age. Many doctors think that if they mention

---

[3]National Institute on Aging, 1991, "Safe Use of Medicines by Older People," *Bound for Good Health,* Washington, D.C.: U.S. Government Printing Office.

the side effects, patients won't take the medicine. Let your doctor know if a drug makes you feel worse. If necessary to get her attention, tell the doctor that the drug's side effects are worse than ever. Have your doctor update the dosages on drugs you've been taking for a long time. Also, listen to your family members. People living with you may notice an adverse drug reaction more quickly than you will. Everyone reacts to drugs differently, and it's up to you to tell your doctor what is happening. Your pharmacist may know more than your doctor on the subject of drugs, so check with him as well.

These are the problems seniors face when becoming health-care consumers. Speak up for yourself! Tell the doctor what kind of treatment you want! In a survey of doctors, patients, and their families, patients said their doctors and loved ones would know what they wanted done if they became demented and then had a heart attack. But their doctors were wrong half the time, and the patients' families didn't do much better.

Options for Long-Term Care

As mentioned earlier, with advancing age comes an increased tendency to experience illnesses of various kinds. These illnesses can eventually result in a need to depend more heavily on others. Such loss of independence and of personal control can be one of the greatest traumas of getting old. It is at this stage that seniors or their family members may begin to consider alternative living situations.

The phrase "long-term care" leads people to think immediately of nursing homes, but there are many other choices to consider. Analyze the situation thoroughly. How much medical care is required? Is ongoing physical therapy needed? What kind of nonmedical care seems necessary? Is a cook, housekeeper, or companion required, or just someone to keep an eye on things?

The options are many: home health care, retirement communities, assisted living facilities, and life care facilities. When more medical attention is required, there are facilities that offer various levels of care. Research the right living situation in the same way you searched for a new doctor.

Talk to others who have already made decisions about long-term care, or ask for help from family and friends. Ask for references from family doctors, the social services administrator at your local hospital, area agencies on aging, and senior centers and organizations. Instead of asking people to recommend a specific place, ask for the names of a couple of places you should check out. Is the facility connected to a hospital? Is it part of a national chain? Is it a nonprofit or charitable institution? Is the care Medicare approved? This might not be necessary now, but it could be later. Is the facility state licensed? What were the results of any state and federal inspection reports? None of this information is confidential, and all of it is readily available to anyone willing to do the research.

You can call the American Association of Retired Persons (AARP) at (800) 424-3410 and request its pamphlet on long-term care for additional information.

Home Health Care

Maybe live-in care isn't required for your situation. Home health care can include help from short-term companions or occasional visits from nurses and other medical professionals. Maybe you could live with other family members: children, brothers, sisters, or grandchildren.

Additional programs that are available include Meals on Wheels, adult day care, senior centers, and respite care, which gives time off to caregivers. You can also get help from escort and transportation services that offer shuttles to doctors' offices. Contact a local AARP office or area agency on aging for additional information.

Retirement Community

Retirement communities are springing up all over the country. They are primarily independent living communities for people, fifty-five years old and above. Everyone owns his own home or condo. There are rules and restrictions that must be followed. The primary one is that all residents must be ambulatory. This is due to fire codes that require residents to be able to evacuate the building on their own. Newer retirement communities are being built within walking distance of college campuses. Besides attending entertainment programs and using the recreational facilities available at a college, seniors can enroll in college courses.

Assisted Living Facility

Assisted living facilities are meant for those who are no longer able to maintain their own homes but are still able to get around on their own. In these facilities, the residents live in their own apartments, which may or may not include a kitchen. Usually at least two meals a day are provided in a community dining room. Residents may come and go as they please. Daily activities are planned for those who are interested. In each apartment there is a call button to be used when emergency help is needed, and there is usually an intermediate care facility on the premises.

Convalescent (Nursing) Home

There is still a need for convalescent or nursing homes. These are live-in health-care facilities, and additional questions need to be asked about them. Is the facility located in a safe area? Are there any restrictions on visitors? Can you leave the facility for walks or visits with friends and family? How many beds are there? How many residents? What are the public areas like? Is there much chance for privacy? What kind of activities are offered? Are social needs met? Are the rules flexible? Who has control over your medications like sedatives and pain relievers? Do you have the right to refuse medication? Avoid places that use restraints to "manage" patients. Make sure that family members and your doctor are notified whenever psychotropic (mind-altering) drugs are given.

The best way to find out whether a place is really good or is just giving you a good sales pitch is to speak to the residents. Ask about the personnel. How many are there? Is there a big turnover? Are they attentive? Do the aides speak English? Do residents have easy access to doctors? Don't ask how the food is; eat there—and not during "visitors'" meals. Is it okay to have food in your room? How do you get food between meals? Remember that for a small facility to run efficiently, residents should all need a similar level of care.

Life Care Facility

A new and increasingly popular option is the life care facility. This form of long-term care allows the resident to stay in the same facility even though personal and medical needs change. As more medical care is required, you are moved into the medical section of the facility. This way, you don't have to keep moving from one facility to another. But there are some drawbacks. Besides an extremely complicated contract, *which should be read by a lawyer,* a large "buy-in" is usually required. This down payment is actually an entrance fee. Understand that most life care facilities don't allow you to sell your membership because you don't own anything, so you may have a problem getting out if you don't like it. There are other things to consider as well. Is your investment secure? Will the company go out of business? What is the quality of medical care being provided? As with all other aspects of health care, the health-care consumer needs to ask questions and make decisions wisely.

Making Medicare Work

What do you think it's like dealing with the federal government on an ongoing basis? Once your medical bills are being paid by Medicare instead of by standard health insurance, you'll find out. First of all, Medicare will not pay all of your health-care costs. Medicare pays only for specific tests, procedures, and doctors' visits. What can you do to minimize your out-of-pocket payments?

Make sure that your doctor accepts Medicare assignment. That means your doctor will accept Medicare's reimbursement, plus your copayment of 20 percent, *as payment in full.* Some doctors will not accept Medicare assignment and expect you to pay all charges above Medicare's "usual and customary" charges. As with all other aspects of health care, remember that this is negotiable. If your doctor refuses to accept Medicare assignment, federal law limits her charges to 115 percent of Medicare's approved amount. Some doctors are getting around these restrictions by charging separately for phone calls, prescription refills, and medical conferences. If your doctor is charging you for these services, remind her that these charges are to be included with the cost of normal office visits.

You may find it difficult to find a doctor who wants to deal with Medicare. Some people think it is illegal for a doctor to refuse to treat a patient covered by Medicare, but this is not true. Like every other member of the business community, the doctor has the right to refuse service to anyone.

So, what do you do? Talk to your current doctor and ask if she accepts Medicare assignment. Most doctors who have been seeing you on an ongoing basis will probably continue to treat you when you become eligible for Medicare. But when interviewing a new doctor, ask specifically if she will accept Medicare assignment. Also, ask if she treats Medicare patients any differently from her other patients.

Some doctors *do* treat Medicare patients differently from those who have private health insurance. In some instances, the doctor may allow a fifteen-minute appointment for Medicare patients and a half-hour for private insurance patients. This is certainly not the case with all doctors, but it does happen. If you feel you are not getting the quality of care you need, tell the doctor. Ask if she would prefer that you look for another doctor to treat you. The doctor may not even realize that she is not meeting your needs. It is important that you discuss the situation with her and then decide what you want to do.

Supplemental Insurance Policies

Even when your doctors accept Medicare assignment, Medicare coverage is often inadequate. "Medigap" insurance policies pay for services not included under Medicare. When shopping around for one of these policies, check the coverage that will be provided to be sure you do not duplicate what you already have.

Covering the Costs of Long-Term Care

Medicare does *not* cover the astronomical costs of long-term nursing home care. Long-term-care insurance is in itself extremely expensive. However, a new long-term-care policy, currently available in New York and Connecticut, and soon to be available in California and Indiana, is provided by insurance companies in partnership with state governments. This new type of policy pays for three years; then Medicaid takes over. The partnership plan costs about one-third less than standard coverage.

There are drawbacks to this new coverage, though. It's only valid in the state where it was purchased. If you live in Connecticut and then move to Massachusetts, it won't help you. Also, the policy only protects your assets, not your income.

Medicare HMOs

Be careful of companies that promote Medicare HMOs. These may be more trouble than they're worth. Most Medicare HMOs, like most other HMOs, require you to choose from a selected group of doctors. But, if you are out of town and need to see a doctor who is not in your group, your treatment may not be covered. If you decide to return to regular Medicare coverage, you may find yourself with no coverage during the crossover period.

Problems with Medicare

Your biggest problems will come from dealing with Medicare itself. Many Medicare claims are rejected as "medically unnecessary." As I pointed out in Chapter 6, high school graduates with *no* medical training make nine-tenths of the decisions on whether Medicare claims should be rejected. Furthermore, *where you live* may determine whether the care you receive is deemed necessary. Medicare decisions vary across the country. Blood tests, for instance, are allowed more often in California than in Illinois. X rays are found necessary more frequently in Wisconsin. Nothing about Medicare is logical. *Always* expect to challenge Medicare's decisions not to pay or to pay less than the amount of the claim. In 1991, more than 50 percent of these decisions were reversed at each appeal level.

There is a Medicare law that states that a patient is not responsible for any bills deemed medically unnecessary unless the patient's doctor

- Has informed her in writing that Medicare may not cover a procedure
- Has provided the reason why it may not be covered
- Has had that patient agree, in writing, to pay the bill[4]

Before you pay any money out of pocket, investigate all the alternatives available. Sometimes the only reason for rejection of a claim is lack of documentation. So *save everything!* Whenever you receive medical bills, make copies for your own files. Write on the back of them why you went to the doctor and what was done. This way if these

---

[4]Joan Harkins, "Questions Asked Most About Medicare," *Good Housekeeping,* March 1995, p. 207.

bills are challenged you will have a record of what services were provided.

These kinds of problems won't faze the informed health-care consumer who knows that nothing good comes easily. If you don't stand up for your needs, no one else will. And it's certainly worth the trouble to get what you need from your doctor.

Chapter 10

Children's Health Care

In pediatric medicine the doctor-patient relationship is more complex than usual because it involves a three-way relationship between doctor, patient, and parents. It is the responsibility of the parents to look out for the best interests of their child. It is the responsibility of the doctor to maintain a relationship with the parents as well as the child. Since doctor and parents both have the common goal of keeping the child healthy, this should not be an impossible task. But it will be more of a challenge than other doctor-patient relationships.

Choosing a Doctor for Your Child

Chapter 2 gave suggestions for choosing a good doctor for your child. Pediatricians are not the only doctors who treat children. You might want to consider family doctors and general practitioners as well; however, family doctors and general practitioners receive only a few months' training in pediatrics, whereas pediatricians have a three-year residency. In rural areas, the population is usually not large enough to support a pediatrician, and family doctors and general practitioners are involved in the total care of the patient and the family.

If you are now pregnant, you will want to choose a doctor for your child before the baby is born. Ask your

OB-GYN to make recommendations. In my search for a pediatrician, I brought in my insurance company's list of approved doctors and asked my OB-GYN to choose from the list. You will also want to talk with friends and family members and see what their suggestions are.

Your health insurance coverage is especially important in the care you provide for your child. Some plans, primarily managed care, include "well-baby" visits at no additional charge. If your insurance coverage doesn't include well-baby visits, the charges can add up to a substantial sum during the first few years. Complete physicals and immunizations are required every year for admittance to schools and day care centers. They are expensive, and it is helpful if they are covered by your health insurance.

Get-Acquainted Visit

Since the initial doctor-patient relationship will be between you and the pediatrician, it is important for the two of you to get to know each other. Schedule a get-acquainted appointment with the pediatrician. Meeting the doctor's staff and seeing his office procedure firsthand is vital. In this doctor-patient relationship you will have just as much interaction with the doctor's staff as with the doctor. Some of the specific issues you will want addressed are

- Whether the office is hectic and out of control.
- Whether the doctor's views mesh with your own.
- Whether the office is properly equipped to handle emergencies. Is portable oxygen available? Are all staff members trained in basic life support?
- Whether there are separate appointment times for well and sick children. Some doctors schedule well-baby appointments in the morning and

non-emergency illness appointments in the afternoon so that diseases aren't passed around the
waiting room.
- Whether there are separate facilities for infectious
children.

Besides learning the doctor's views on health care in
general, you will want to tell the doctor about your family's medical background. It was important for the doctor
to know that I had cancer while I was pregnant and to discuss with me the potential impact on my child's health.

By choosing a doctor for your baby before it is born,
you will assure that your baby gets the care that is needed
at the time of delivery. When you are admitted to the hospital to give birth, the staff will inform the pediatrician so
that he or another doctor from his office can be there to
check the baby. You will also know in advance what appointments are necessary for the care of your newborn.

If you are changing pediatricians and your child is not
a newborn, ask how many patients of your child's age the
doctor treats. If your child is thirteen years old, you will
not want to take him to a doctor who specializes in kids
under ten. Some pediatricians have a subspecialty in adolescent medicine. This may be a good choice for your
child. An older child should be involved in the interviewing process as well.

Treating the Child and the Family

A good pediatrician considers the whole family when
she is treating the child. When it was time for my daughter to start her polio vaccinations, I was undergoing radiation therapy. My daughter's doctor informed me that, since
my immune system was compromised by the radiation,

polio could be transmitted to me by the live virus that would be injected into my daughter. She vaccinated my daughter with the inactive virus. It was very important that our pediatrician knew the specific health problems in our family and considered our special needs.

Sometimes the pediatrician's concern for our family has saved us money. My daughter was diagnosed with strep throat when my husband also had a bad sore throat. As usual, he had been putting off going to the doctor to have it checked out. The pediatrician's nurse suggested that he call his doctor to say our daughter had a confirmed case of strep throat and that he had a sore throat as well. She said his doctor would probably prescribe antibiotics for him without seeing him first. He did.

Doctors are not the only health-care professionals who care for children. Many pediatricians' offices employ nurse practitioners. These professionals have taken medical classes that give them extended responsibilities in their jobs. They practice under a doctor's supervision and in many states are qualified to write prescriptions. Many doctors believe nurse practitioners will become more responsible for hands-on health care in the future.

When to Call Your Child's Doctor

New parents usually have many questions about how to care for their newborn. Parents of older children frequently have concerns because they know that kids can get very sick very quickly. When is it appropriate to call the doctor with questions about your child's health?

Most doctors will tell you that they would rather have you call with questions than ignore a potentially serious situation. How will *you* know if you should call? First, ask your doctor to recommend a good general information book on children's health care. Reading this book will let you know what to expect as your child grows up. It will describe how to deal with drooling, teething, crying, and temper tantrums. It will tell you when the baby should be lifting his head, rolling over, crawling, walking, and talking. You will learn that there's nothing to be concerned about when your child is one year old and not yet toilet trained even though everyone you know has told you that *their* child was toilet trained at nine months.

At times you will need to call the doctor's office after hours. Don't be afraid to call with an emergency, no matter what the time of day. When you call, let the answering service know it is an emergency and ask when you can expect a call back. Many doctors pick up their calls once an hour. If this is not soon enough, let the answering service know that you need a call back as soon as possible. If your doctor or the doctor on call does not respond in ten minutes, call again. Be aware that the answering service is not staffed by nurses; they're telephone operators with no medical training. You may need to be persistent. Call your doctor if

- Your child is over six months old and has a temperature of 102 degrees or higher
- Your child has a fever that lasts more than three days or rises abruptly
- Your child is rubbing and scratching his ear and is cranky or in pain; also if there is a discharge from the ear
- Your child has a severe sore throat
- Your child is acting "different"
- Your child is not sleeping through the night and has abdominal pain
- Your child has difficulty breathing

- A cold lasts more than ten to fourteen days
- You're not sure how much medicine to give to your child
- *Any* time you're uncertain or worried

Trust *your* feelings about when you should call your child's doctor.

The Problem Parent

The most common complaint of pediatricians is that parents forget to use common sense. One job of pediatricians is teaching parents to trust their instincts in caring for their children.

Not all parents feel competent in dealing with their child's problems. They become dependent on their doctor's advice. Should you be concerned that you are one of these parents? Ask yourself these questions.

- Are you calling the doctor daily?
- Are you asking questions that aren't health related, like "What kind of birthday cake do you give a one-year-old?"
- Do you refuse to make any decision concerning your child unless you've checked it out with the doctor first?
- Are you calling the doctor in the middle of the night with problems that could have been handled during the day?

If these symptoms sound like yours, you might want to reconsider your doctor-patient-parent relationship and begin to take more responsibility.

Of course, this doesn't mean you shouldn't call your child's doctor when something doesn't seem right. Perhaps your child has a rash you've never seen before, or she's not acting the way she usually does. By all means, you should call the doctor then.

Appropriate Emergency Care

Children run hard, play hard, and have no fear. Her very nature almost guarantees that your child will have to go to an emergency room at some point in her life. Ideally, all pediatric health care should be carried out at facilities that specialize in caring for children. This is especially true in emergencies, but such specialized care is not always available. In the United States there are over five thousand general emergency rooms but only about sixty pediatric emergency departments.

Make a list of the medicines your child is currently taking. List your child's known allergies to medicines *and* foods. If your child is allergic to seafood, she will probably also be allergic to iodine; this is important to know in an emergency. Take this list with you to the emergency room. If your child is in day care or in someone else's care, make sure her caregivers have a copy of this list. You should also give them a signed authorization letter allowing them to consent to emergency care for your child.

Pediatricians in the Emergency Room

Before you need to use an emergency room, ask your doctor which one in your area you should have your child taken to. Only a small percentage of general emergency departments have pediatricians or pediatric emergency physicians on staff. Child-size equipment is not widely available either.

Although children are generally treated like adults in emergency situations, they shouldn't be. Children need to be treated sooner, within the first half-hour of any emergency. Children's reactions to injuries are different from adults'. They are more vulnerable to head injury, less tolerant of blood loss, and have greater risk of breathing problems. Also, drug dosages for children are different from those for adults. If emergency room doctors don't know these special needs and don't have the training and equipment to treat children, an emergency can become life threatening for your child.

Your pediatrician is probably on staff at a hospital with an emergency room that does have the necessary care and equipment available for your child. Confirm where your child should be taken in an emergency.

Care in the Ambulance

The care of children in ambulances is of concern as well. EMTs (emergency medical technicians) receive extremely limited training in pediatrics, only three hours out of a hundred. Child-size oxygen masks and blood pressure cuffs are rarely available. Children need airway tubes less than half the width of those for adults. Talk to ambulance companies in your area to decide which one you should call in an emergency. If you are calling the operator or 911 with an emergency involving a child, request a properly equipped ambulance service.

Demand Quality Emergency Care

If the shortcomings described in the preceding section were present in adult emergency services, they would never be allowed to continue. But children don't vote and they have no political voice. Most parents and guardians have been under the mistaken impression that there was nothing to worry about. Now that you know differently, demand better emergency care for children. Ask your child's doctor what *you* can do to improve the pediatric emergency care situation. Call your health insurance company and make its staff aware of your concerns. Talk to your local hospitals and ambulance companies. If they are not equipped to handle children's emergencies, let them know you will use hospitals and ambulances that are so equipped. Complain, cajole, insist, and demand! Use your consumer clout to get your children the quality emergency care they deserve.

Making Young Adults Responsible for Their Own Care

Besides providing your child with the quality health care he needs, you are setting an example for your child in how to carry on a doctor–health-care consumer relationship. Many parents find they're far more demanding about care for their children than they are about their own care. When parents demand and get better care for their children, it tends to make them more vigilant in their own health-care matters.

During your child's medical appointments, see that there is good communication between the doctor and your child. As your child grows older, have him talk directly to the doctor about his concerns and the treatments available. If he's not sure about something, have him talk to the doctor directly and not rely on you as an intermediary. If the doctor views this as a waste of his time, *find a new doctor.* You will not always be responsible for obtaining health care for your child. After age fifteen or sixteen, depending on where you live, your child can seek independent medical care without your approval. He will also have the right to refuse treatment. When this time comes, you want to be sure your child knows how to act as a vigilant health-care consumer on his own behalf.

When Children Control Their Health-Care Needs

Your goal as a parent is to teach your children to be health-care consumers. You will also want to help them get to know their bodies. Teach them to recognize when they're coming down with a cold, not getting enough sleep, or eating too much sugar. As they become adolescents, they will probably want to take more responsibility for their health-care choices and decisions.

Privacy is important to adolescents, and your child will not want you to be as involved in her health care as you have been. If she has a chronic condition like asthma or diabetes, she'll have to learn how to deal with her illness in everyday situations. The doctor–health-care consumer relationship becomes extremely important here. Even if you have discussed adolescent health issues with your child, she may want to get a "second opinion" from her doctor.

Cigarettes, drugs, alcohol, and sex are all easily accessible to teenagers. They may not want to discuss their use or nonuse with you, but let them know that they can discuss these topics with a doctor. If they would prefer to talk with another doctor, have them ask their pediatrician for a referral to someone who has experience in those areas.

A parent will not always be able to find out what is happening with his child's health-care needs at this point.

If the child asks her doctor for complete confidentiality, that will include her parents. And the doctor must comply. If the doctor–health-care consumer team has been built up over the years, your child's health-care needs will more easily be met even though you may be excluded.

There are some health situations that commonly cause concern during the adolescent years; depression, eating disorders, and anxiety are some of them. Not everyone has these problems, but if you think your child may be affected, discuss your concerns with your child's doctor.

Changes in Established Treatments

You need to be active in your child's health care for as long as he allows you to be. Medicine changes constantly; new information is released, prescribed treatments are revised, and widely accepted treatments are questioned.

Some of the newest information includes the following.

- Measles as a health threat is back again. Ask your doctor if your child needs a second vaccine.
- A single injection of an antibiotic to treat ear infections can be as effective as ten days of oral antibiotics.
- Children of smokers are twice as likely as children of nonsmokers to develop asthma.
- Children who stutter are *not* likely to outgrow the problem without therapy.
- Lead poisoning affects one out of six children in the United States.
- Tonsillectomies are not the wonder cure for recurring ear and throat infections, as once was thought.

- Back problems in teens need to be treated more aggressively than in adults. A wait-and-see approach may make the problems worse.

And don't forget the most important question of all, "What happens if we just wait?"

Keep up to date on what is being discovered about children's illnesses and treatments. When you are confronted with information you aren't sure about, ask questions. Is this the current standard of care for this condition? And don't forget the most important question of all, "What happens if we just wait?"

Until your child is old enough to speak up for himself and his health-care needs, it is up to you to act on his behalf. When your child is old enough, teach him to speak up for himself. Let him know that this is how he will get the quality health care he deserves.

Chapter 11

Buyer Beware

In Chapter 1, Rule 3 was "Medicine is a business." This chapter will focus on the business of medicine: how it affects you and what you can do to see that you receive the quality care you require.

Managed Care

Most doctors agree that managed care provided through an HMO is the future of health care. Approximately 96 percent of people covered by employer-provided health-care plans are enrolled in managed care or preferred provider plans. Both arrangements restrict the choice of doctors to those on the insurance plan's list.

Managed care is not "commonsense" care. It is turning out to be health care for the masses, literally. If you go to an HMO doctor during flu season, you can expect to find a waiting room full of patients and you may have a long wait ahead of you. If you have something serious, the doctor may tell you to wait and see. At times tests that should be done immediately may be postponed. Managed care was designed to lower health-care costs and improve the quality of care. But you may find yourself having to fight to get that quality care. If it becomes necessary, stand up for your needs and insist on the health-care you require.

HMOs do a great deal of high-profile marketing. You can watch their television commercials and hear how great HMOs are: "Choose your own doctor. Get the care you need when you need it." The health-care consumer knows that these statements are puffery put out by advertising departments and may have little or nothing to do with the actual service.

Check out specific health insurance plans before you sign up. Ask about complaints from patients. What about patient satisfaction and doctor turnover? What kind of choice *do* you have in this plan? Will these details be put in writing? Can you change doctors if you're not satisfied with your first choice? Does the insurance company qualify its network doctors on the basis of experience as well as on their agreeing to price constraints?

Many HMO companies will not discuss specifics of their plans because they see this as proprietary information. This stance may be fine in other businesses, but in health care, your life is on the line.

What kind of information won't HMO companies divulge? *New York* magazine stated that U.S. Healthcare in New York State refused to say which hospitals were part of its HMO network in Manhattan. And the company wouldn't be specific about how many of its internists in Manhattan were board certified.[1] These are important questions whose answers indicate the quality of care you can expect. If you can't get the information you need to make an informed choice, don't join that HMO. Remember, companies put their best foot forward to make a sale. If one won't answer your concerns *before* you join, you can be sure it won't cooperate once you're a member.

---

[1]Jeanne Kassler, "Managed Care—Or Chaos?" *New York* magazine, August 23, 1993, p. 49.

HMOs make their money on the number of people who sign up. Once you've signed up, the company will do all it can to *save* money, not spend it.

Rationed Care

Managed-care companies will be the first to tell you that they do not ration care. They just make sure that they save money on excessive and expensive care. Unfortunately, what one person sees as excessive another may view as necessary. Find out what incentives are being given to limit the care provided.

In most HMOs, doctors are paid a per-patient, or capitation, fee. The doctor is paid a set amount, determined by the patient's age, for each patient's care per month. No matter how often you see your primary doctor that month, the doctor will get paid the same amount. This amount also covers any referrals your doctor gives you for specialists, tests, or procedures. At the end of the year, if the doctor has not spent all the money designated for his patients' care, he is eligible for a bonus.

Choose your doctor carefully. Your doctor will be your advocate with the health insurance company. If you have concerns regarding where your doctor's allegiance lies, ask him how he handles the inherent problems in making more money when he provides less care.

Quality Care

It *is* possible to receive quality care from HMOs. But you need to educate yourself. Go to free health seminars and watch health-care specials on television. News shows are constantly spotlighting different medical procedures, treatments, and cures. Know what screening tests are recommended for your age group and be sure you discuss these with your doctor.

Be insistent and persistent. Don't take no for an answer. If you're not happy, *complain*. Complain to your employer, your doctor, and the management of the HMO. The answer you'll probably get is, "That's just the way it is." Don't believe it! Most complaints that go through the proper channels for settlement of grievances are settled in favor of the patient. Sometimes saying no is just a way of weeding out those who don't want to spend the time and energy to reach a *yes*. The health-care consumer knows that the extra time and energy are well worth the end result.

Many doctors feel that in the future managed-care companies will be held responsible for the quality of care they deliver. In 1993 a jury ordered an HMO to pay more than $12 million to the estate of a woman who was refused a bone marrow transplant as treatment for her breast cancer. A *Wall Street Journal* article said that the jury found the HMO had acted in bad faith, breached its contract, and recklessly inflicted emotional distress. It also noted that the executive who had decided not to cover the procedure was given bonuses when he saved the company money.[2]

This does not mean that you are in a hopeless situation if your health-care insurance is with a managed-care company. Besides following the suggestions in Chapter 2 on finding the best doctor for you, here are a few other things you should do.

---

[2]Ellen Joan Pollack, "HMO Held Liable for Refusing Coverage," *Wall Street Journal,* December 28, 1993, p. B4.

- Ask if your doctor is on the HMO's board. If he is, he will have greater control over decisions in getting you the care you need.
- If you're not satisfied with the care you receive, ask for a second opinion from another in-network doctor. Ask for an out-of-network doctor's opinion if you feel that monetary concerns are taking precedence over your health-care needs.
- If you are scheduled to have a procedure done, find out what kind of experience the doctor has with that procedure. If the in-network doctor does not have the necessary experience, or if you require very specialized care that is not available in your HMO, ask for your care to be provided by an out-of-network doctor. HMOs *do* approve out-of-network treatment, but only when a patient insists.
- Compare the health care you receive with that of family and friends. If there are significant differences, find out why.

HMOs and managed-care companies are now aggressively trying to persuade seniors to sign up for their services. Employers are also recommending HMOs to their retirees to save on costs. But is this a good option? Most seniors in this situation would have to switch from their current doctor to a doctor on the plan. Making a change could be a problem for those with chronic illnesses. Seniors seem to get better care with standard Medicare and "Medigap" policies, which allow them to continue their ongoing relationship with their own doctor.

The health-care consumer can get the care he needs from HMOs and managed care. Insist, demand, and argue.

The squeaky wheel is definitely the one that gets the attention in managed-care situations. An HMO executive once told me that people just don't realize that companies *have* to hold costs down so that they can make money. On the contrary, I think we all understand that. But I think we also all believe that companies should offer excellent service while they're making money.

The Business of Selling Medicine

Over-the-Counter Products

Go to your local drugstore and you will be amazed to see what is available in OTC treatments. People use these medicines much of the time to treat themselves without a doctor's help. However, there is a general misperception that all medicines or treatments sold over the counter are less potent than prescription treatments. This is not true. Take aspirin, for example. Aspirin has been used to prevent heart attacks and migraine headaches. Some researchers believe that aspirin can prevent certain kinds of cancer. And doctors recommend aspirin for some people suffering from dementia. But for all the good aspirin does, it should not be taken indiscriminately. Aspirin can cause bleeding ulcers and is not recommended for pregnant women because the effects on the baby are unknown and it may cause excessive bleeding during childbirth.

Every year, drugs that were previously sold by prescription only are put out in OTC form. This is not done for the public good. It is done because drug companies know that greater accessibility to the general public means better sales potential. Once a drug is approved for OTC sale, a company will spend a lot of money to introduce the drug to the public. In the past few years, you have probably heard about Motrin, Gyne-Lotrimin, and Tavist. Not only have you heard about them, you have seen full-page magazine ads, as well as coupons so you could try them at a reduced price.

But what else do you know about these drugs? What conditions do they treat? How much should you take, and how often? Is it all right for you to take these drugs with your other medications? Should certain foods not be eaten while this medication is being taken? These are important questions to ask when you are considering a new medication. Your doctor can tell you why he is prescribing a prescription drug and can give you appropriate dosage information, as well as any other necessary information. With OTC medicines, you make the decisions. Ask for help from your doctor and pharmacist in making these decisions about taking OTC medicines. Did you know that the FDA doesn't require drug manufacturers to test drugs on children before they are put on the market? As a result, there's really no way of knowing what dose is appropriate or effective for children. That's why the bottles always tell parents to consult a physician.

Over-the-Counter Tests You can find out when you're ovulating or if you're pregnant. If you want to know what your blood sugar level is, there's a test for that. You can monitor your blood pressure and listen to your heartbeat. If you want to know what your cholesterol level is or whether you have a urinary tract infection, you can buy the available tests and follow directions. But before you do the testing, think about what you will do with the results once you have them. Will you make the treatment decisions yourself or will you confirm the answers with your doctor?

When you use a test, make sure you do so properly. Read *all* the instructions *before* you begin the test. Follow the directions exactly and be sure that the test is performed under as sterile conditions as possible. Be aware that the results you receive from these tests will not be as accurate as those from your doctor's office or a lab.

Some drug companies are considering selling home tests for sexually transmitted diseases such as AIDS, gonorrhea, and chlamydia. Doctors are concerned. They are afraid that members of the public will not get the follow-up care they may need from their health-care providers. Instead, individuals may try to treat themselves with left-over medicine or skip treatment altogether, resulting in serious complications and in the further spread of these diseases.

Over-the-Counter Treatments There are over 100,000 nonprescription products in the marketplace. Consumers can choose from medicines, sprays, ointments, and medical devices that claim to address a dazzling array of problems and ills. And don't forget vitamins! Just some of the supplements you'll find are iron, niacin, garlic, ginsing, zinc, calcium, beta-carotene, folic acid, and antioxidants. Make sure your doctor is aware of any over-the-counter treatments, including vitamins and supplements, that you are taking, as well as the dosages. Some of these products can cause side effects when too much is taken or when they mix with other drugs you are taking.

Many medical devices are also available without prescription. If you hurt your neck or back, you can buy a cervical collar. You can also purchase back supports, arm slings, hinged knee braces, wrist braces, canes, and crutches. Be aware, though, that if you are contemplating using these products, you might want to schedule a doctor's appointment first to rule out anything serious.

There are also products of an intimate nature. For birth control, contraceptive foam, contraceptive sponges, bio-adhesive contraceptive gel, the female condom, and men's condoms with various attributes are all available. There's even the Stop Bedwetting Kit should you need to deal with that problem.

Homeopathic remedies are also available including, for example, an arthritis formula, one to stop smoking, and treatments for allergies, colds, and the flu.

If you are prone to allergies, you should be careful whenever using any over-the-counter treatments. Do you know what's in that cold/flu/sinus medication you're taking? What are the ingredients in that sleeping preparation? And, of course, don't underestimate the cost. Few of these treatments come cheap; some may cost as much as one hundred dollars.

The Problems of Self-Diagnosis

Many people argue that the public's access to all these medical tests and treatments is a good thing. They say it's important to have control of your health-care needs so you don't have to rely on your doctor for every little concern. Unfortunately, when you are treating yourself, there is a lot of room for error.

Are you treating symptoms and ignoring an underlying illness? Let's say you haven't been feeling well lately. You're very tired, and you've been dizzy and nauseous. A friend thinks you might be pregnant, so you buy a home pregnancy test at the supermarket. You take the test and are thrilled when it turns up negative. But what do you do now? Do you go to the doctor to see why you're not feeling well? If you're like most people, you just ignore the situation, thinking you've done your part in searching out the cause. Six months later when you're *really* not doing well, you finally go to the doctor.

This is not to say that sometimes a cold is not just a cold. You take your pain reliever and cough drops and you get better. But do you know the dangers of taking those over-the-counter medicines? The FDA certifies that OTC drugs are safe and effective *when taken according to directions*. Did you know that if you take more than the recommended dosage of acetaminophen or take it on an empty stomach or with alcohol, you could have severe liver or kidney damage? This is important information for those who believe that "if two pills work, four pills will work even better."

If you read the warning label on many brands of cough drops you will see that you should use them for no more than two days at a time. And you should be taking only one every two hours. Is that how *you* take cough drops?

If you are *always* using some kind of over-the-counter medicine, discuss this practice with your doctor. Make sure that what you are treating are just simple problems, like tension headache or indigestion. If the same problem keeps recurring, perhaps there is an underlying condition you should have checked out.

Be the health-care consumer you need to be. OTC treatments are not always the most effective or cost-efficient way of dealing with a health concern. Ask your pharmacist what she recommends. She will be able to confirm that the medicine you choose will not conflict with any other drugs you're currently taking. If you treat yourself and the problem has not cleared up in a couple of days, *call your doctor.* Tell him what you've done so far and ask what he thinks the next step should be.

Other Health-Care Consumer Issues

There are many other situations the health-care consumer may need to handle. Just remember, you are being approached as a customer. As long as you realize this, you will be able to make the proper choices.

Pharmacies

Managed care has made an impact on the quality of your doctor's care, and it seems to be affecting pharmacies as well. In order to get the business of HMOs, pharmacies have lowered the cost of their drugs. They intend to make up that money by filling a greater number of prescriptions. Pharmacists now have to fill more prescriptions than ever before. With the increase in prescriptions comes a greater chance of errors being made.

Once, I discovered that my prescription for antihistamines had been filled incorrectly with painkillers. Now, whenever I get a new prescription, I look it up in the *Physician's Desk Reference (PDR)* to make sure I've received the correct medication. The *PDR* is the book doctors use to decide which medication to prescribe. The book includes pictures of most of the drugs manufactured in the United States and descriptions of their uses and their side effects. You should confirm with the pharmacist the directions for usage. How many pills do you take, how often, and for how long? Mistakes do happen, so be aware of what you're taking and check every prescription you get.

Injuries at Work

If you are injured at work, you will most likely be sent to a company doctor who deals with workers' compensation claims. Since this is likely to be an emergency situation, you will not be able to research the doctor's qualifications. Make sure that she knows the general state of your health, and tell her the name of your regular doctor. Ask her to keep your doctor up to date on your situation.

Tell the doctor and the staff of any allergies you have. If you haven't had a tetanus shot in a while, ask if you need one now.

If you want to confirm the company doctor's diagnosis, call your own doctor and tell him the situation. Ask your doctor if there is any treatment he would recommend in your situation. Tell your personnel department if you feel you are not getting adequate care from the company doctor. Let the personnel department staff members know that you will be holding them personally responsible for the quality of care that you receive, since they have chosen the health-care provider.

Direct Mail Solicitations

Health-care companies, like all other businesses, are finding it continually harder to make money. This includes health-care charities that depend on donations from the public. Like any other business, many of them are purchasing mailing lists so they can target the people most likely to donate to their cause.

When I got home from the hospital with my newborn daughter, I found a solicitation from a foundation raising money to fight sudden infant death syndrome. They requested a donation "to ensure the continued good health of my newborn child." This foundation must have bought a "new mothers" mailing list.

While I was in radiation treatment for Hodgkin's, I received a direct mail request for a contribution to prevent animals from being used for medical experimentation. The letter expressed outrage that animals were being used to find cures for cancer, epilepsy, and other health problems. Needless to say, this organization had targeted the wrong prospect. I knew firsthand the importance of using animals in medical research.

The business practices these groups employed outraged me. They shouldn't have . . . it was just a case of a business approaching me as a consumer. And I used my consumer clout—I did not donate to these causes. I also told friends and family members about what these foundations did, and they refused to donate, too.

Health-Care Privacy

Most people think that *all* matters between doctor and patient are private. This is not always true. If you have purchased your health insurance through your employer, you can be sure your employer knows everything there is to know about your health. Since employers are the ones paying the bills, they get a copy of every claim.

If your child is sick and the school wants documentation from a doctor stating when he'll be able to return to school, tell the doctor's office to send a letter with only the information requested. If you don't, the office staff might find it more convenient to send a copy of the entire file instead of taking the time to write a letter. There is no reason to pass along your child's medical information to anyone.

In reality, people give others access to their medical files every day. When you apply for a new job, the personnel department may ask to have access to your medical records. Lawyers can subpoena your records if you're involved in any kind of lawsuit. These records come in handy particularly in divorce and custody cases.

Have you ever heard of the Medical Information Bureau (MIB)? This is a clearinghouse of medical information on practically everyone who has ever set foot in a hospital or had lab tests performed. Life insurance and health insurance companies contact the MIB when they are about to insure a new client. Through the MIB's files they are able to check out the applicant's health background and see if there is any reason that they would not want to insure that person.

You may think you have nothing to be worried about. But have you ever had a blood test for AIDS—just as a precaution maybe, or to prove to someone that there was no reason for concern? Is there a history of breast cancer in your family? Did you have a mammogram done at an early age just to make sure you were all right? Have you been treated for depression or a drinking problem? These records in your medical file could stop an insurance company from covering you in the future.

Where does the MIB get its information? From labs, clinics, hospitals, and doctor's offices. Do you smoke? Do you have a great deal of stress in your life? Have you mentioned to your doctor that you occasionally use recreational drugs? All these comments made to your doctor in privacy may be included in your MIB record. Check with *all* your health-care providers and ask if they pass on information to interested parties. If they do, let them know that you don't approve of this practice, and demand that they don't do it to you!

What else can you do? Contact the MIB (617-426-3660) and request a copy of your file. Read through it carefully. If there are errors, make sure you get them corrected.

Look out for your own and your family's interests, and you will ensure that you get what you need from the health-care industry.

Chapter 12

The Future of Health Care

The Changing Landscape of Medicine

Medicine is constantly changing. Our approach to medicine, and health care in general, needs to change too. The family doctor who used to make house calls is gone. He has been replaced by the doctor–health-care consumer team. Preventive health care is taking the place of waiting to see your doctor until you're really sick. Blindly following your doctor's orders has given way to asking questions, researching treatment plans, and jointly deciding on your health-care needs.

Some people find it difficult to meet these new challenges, but they are taking that major step and becoming health-care consumers. Stand up for your needs and keep one eye fixed on the future.

What's New and Different

As long as I can remember, my dad has had a bad back. Twenty-five years ago the doctors tried to talk him into surgery. My dad told them that he would wait until they came out with a pill to fix the problem. The recommended treatment for many back problems today is light exercise and painkillers, not surgery.

There has also been a significant change in thinking when it comes to painkillers. The accepted medical belief in the past was that you had to be careful about patients becoming addicted to painkillers. There was an assumption that pain built character and that it was necessary to learn how to "tough it out." Today we know that a person in pain is unnecessarily stressing his body and actually delaying healing. Doctors are also starting to rethink pain management for terminally ill patients, striving to make their final days pain free.

We used to think there was no danger in smoking. Now we know better. The newest findings include the dangers of passive smoke. Researchers now think that passive smoking may cause lung cancer in those who have never smoked.

Not only are we learning more about the health dangers that have always been around us, we are finding new ways to treat diseases. A new drug called Cognex is being used to treat Alzheimer's disease. This is a big step forward for a disease that was once not only untreatable but undiagnosable until after death.

Research and development are two of the most important factors in the future of health care. Thirty years ago there was no established treatment for Hodgkin's disease. Today Hodgkin's is one of the most curable forms of cancer. Yes, I am a firm believer in research and development! Yet many people see it as the easiest place to cut health-care funding. The results of the monies being spent on research and development are not immediate, but I look forward to the day when a cure will be found for breast cancer, heart disease, and the other deadly illnesses we face every day.

The Food and Drug Administration

It is the job of the Food and Drug Administration (FDA) to test and approve medical products and drugs for use in the United States. The FDA requires that these new products and drugs be proven safe and effective before they are approved. Some drug companies would prefer that the only standard to be met is that of safety. But wouldn't you like to know that the drugs and products you use will be effective? It's hard enough to make the proper choices among products that have been deemed safe and effective. Who wants to make a selection from a shelf full of ineffective but safe choices?

The FDA has also been given tremendous power regarding the *quality* of health-care products. Once the FDA approves a device that is to be injected or implanted—like pacemakers, heart valves, and artificial joints—the manufacturer cannot be sued if there are problems with those products. *Business Week* magazine described a situation with a wrinkle-softening treatment called Zyderm.[1] Several women who had used Zyderm came down with an incurable immune system disease and sued the manufacturer for knowingly marketing an unsafe product. So far, the decisions have been in favor of the manufacturer. A Massachusetts federal appeals court ruled that Congress expects the FDA, not the courts, to be the authority on the safety and effectiveness of medical devices. Manufacturers of health-care products state that this is an important ruling and that freedom from the threat of litigation will result in lower prices for the consumer.

But the health-care consumer knows that price should not be the primary issue in health-care decisions. The public also needs safe, effective, and high-quality products. Write or call the FDA. Let them know that it is important to everyone that quality standards be upheld.

---

[1]"An Invincible Shield for Medical Manufacturers," *Business Week,* August 9, 1993, p. 73.

The Impact of
Genetic Research on the Public

Health care has come a long way toward being able to predict the possibility of getting diseases, thanks to genetic testing. Genetic indicators have been found for breast cancer, colon and rectal cancer, cystic fibrosis, some tumors, and Lou Gehrig's disease. Many people at risk for specific diseases are now forewarned. Maybe in the future we will know if someone is prone to heart disease or Alzheimer's and will begin treatment earlier. But today, these tests only measure the genetic predisposition to certain diseases. Negative findings do not necessarily mean that you won't get a disease.

The Consumer's Right
to Choose

The most important part of being a health-care consumer is knowing that, in all except the most dire emergency situations, you have the time to choose. The health-care consumer knows how to choose the right health insurance plan, the right doctor, the right hospital, and other health-care providers. He knows how to research and evaluate treatment options. And finally, the health-care consumer knows that the doctor–health-care consumer relationship is important to the quality of health care.

The Doctor's Responsibility

After all is said and done, the health-care consumer still must be able to trust and rely on his doctor. For some people, this is just not possible. They have had problems in the past with doctors, and when they tried to work it out, the problems were ignored.

Different methods are being used today to deal with problem doctors. In the past, complaints were most often filed with state medical boards or registered through civil malpractice suits. Today, there's more willingness to press criminal charges and assess jail time. This increase in severity comes, in part, because doctors' peer review groups have not been effective in holding doctors responsible for their actions. Many state medical and disciplinary boards don't punish doctors sufficiently. They may have given a slap on the wrist, but it ended there.

In Chapter 7, I mentioned an OB-GYN whose patients accused him of improper actions that included molestation. Over a ten-year period, complaints had been lodged against him with the local medical boards. But not much was done. Each patient was informed that she was the only one who had complained. Eventually, *some* restrictions were put on the doctor's license, but he was allowed to continue his practice. This situation finally came to an end when several of the women went to the media with their complaints. This doctor is now in criminal court, charged with twenty-seven counts of sexual abuse.

Most doctors will tell you that the "experts in their area" should do the disciplining. But if misconduct ends up being swept under the rug, no one wins. If you detect misconduct, speak up and follow up! First, talk with the doctor directly. If that doesn't help, discuss the situation with another doctor you trust. Contact the hospital the doctor is affiliated with, your health insurance company, and your employer. Most importantly, remember that *you* did not cause the situation. You are not at fault.

The Responsibility of the Health-Care Consumer

Guilt seems to play a big part in health care. People are always feeling as though they should have known better. They blame themselves for getting sick and for not getting care when they need it. This is particularly true for people with cancer. We are told the warning signs of cancer, how to prevent it, how to eat healthy, exercise, and give ourselves self-examinations. Still, people are diagnosed with cancer every day.

Guilt has no place in health care. Doctors are finding that even the healthiest people living the healthiest lifestyles can still come down with life-threatening illnesses. The purpose of this book is to give you the skills necessary to research and find the quality health care that you and your family deserve. I hope that it has also shown you that you don't have to accept the answer, "That's just the way it's done." A close friend of mine once told me that I always saw "rules and procedures" as something meant for others, not for me. I guess that's true. I don't accept the status quo—things can *always* be better. That's the outlook you need to have. Strive for the best health care possible. Work with your doctor as a team. His knowledge and experience, along with your determination and perseverance, will get you the quality care you need.

GOOD LUCK AND GOOD HEALTH!